Art and Spiritual Growth

Chinese Cultural Experiences and Design

中华文化创意丛书

艺术与心灵成长

俞鹰 主编

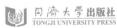

同济大学出版社
TONGJI UNIVERSITY PRESS

宁静而快乐的心态看似无为，但它发送出的信号却能让身体无不为。

A serene and merry mind seems to do nothing, but it sends out signals telling the cells to do everything.

随着我们净化及简化细体，灵魂的喜悦会从内在散发出来，而我们就能够将自己的意识扩展到更高的状态，揭示出越来越多的人类潜能。

As we purify and simplify the subtle body, the joy of the soul radiates from within, and we are able to expand our consciousness into higher states, revealing more and more of our human potential.

我们需要认识的是欲念只会增加不快乐，而零欲望则能无限增加幸福感。在这个状态当中，我们没有任何期盼，不会与自己或他人玩游戏，不会操纵人或对他们有任何期待。

We have to realise that having desires is only going to increase our unhappiness and having zero desires is going to infinitely increase our happiness. In this state, we don't expect anything. When we don't expect anything, we don't play games with ourselves or with others. We don't manipulate others because we don't expect anything from them.

满心能够把我们带到最开始的基础——精神平衡和平静的状态。

Heartfulness can bring us to first base – to a state of mental balance and peace.

序

　　2010年5月，我回到同济大学参加中华文化传播中心的揭牌仪式，与同济大学的师生们共同见证了一个新的中华文化传播平台，一个人文、艺术和科技复合型人才培养基地的诞生。作为五年来中心创造性探索的素描和代表性成果的剪辑，"中华文化创意丛书"很好地展示了同济大学中华文化传播中心的工作及其成效。对于中华文化传播中心在传播和弘扬中华文化，以及创新人才培养方面取得的成绩，我感到欣喜和振奋。

　　随着全球化的加速发展，科技创新能力与文化传播能力成为国家国际竞争力的核心。风靡世界的好莱坞大片和畅销全球的苹果手机，生动诠释了先进科技与流行文化"联手"的巨大威力。中国要由经济大国变成经济强国，从"中国制造"升级为"中国创造"，也需要科技创新和文化传播的比翼齐飞、相得益彰。

　　中华文化博大精深，涵养了丰富的创新元素。神话、哲学、诗歌为人们提供了大量抽象的创新元素，梅兰竹菊、文房四宝、亭台楼阁、桌椅台榻等则为人们提供了大量具象的创新元素。通过发掘、体悟、领会，对中华文化进行创新性发展和创造性转化，让人文、艺术和科技深度融合，内化于心，外显于形，设计和生产出既体现当代科技水平，又能满足人们生活和审美需要的产品，乃是"中国制造"升级之正途，更是"中国创造"发展之真义。

　　当前，世界经济结构和消费结构正在经历快速升级，人们对差异化、个性化产品的需求迅速增长。如果我们能够通过智能科技将中国巨大的生产能力"柔性化"，把根植于中华文化、汲取了世界多元文化之精髓的创意融入个性化设计和小规模定制，将科技的力量、艺术的气息和人文的温热融入产品设计和制造当中，那么，实现由"中国制造"向"中国创造"的转变不再是难事，中华文化和中国科技也会为世界经济发展和人类文明做出更大贡献。

　　大众创业、万众创新的根本是尊重每个人的创新创业权利，发掘每个人的创新创业潜能。鼓励大众创业、万众创新，最重要的是要为更多的人"赋能"，让科技发展的最新成果成为更多人创新创业的平台，让中华文化中的抽象、具象元素启发更多人，让他们能够从艺术、审美和体验出发设计产品，满足人们多样化、多层次的需求。如此，大众创业、万众创新就有了源头活水。

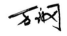

全国政协副主席、科学技术部原部长

Preface

In May, 2010, I went back to Tongji University for the inauguration of the Chinese Cultural Center, and together with all the faculty, I witnessed the birth of a new platform for transmitting Chinese culture, which is dedicated to bringing up comprehensive talents regarding humanity, arts, science and technology. Representing the 5-year creative research of the center, Chinese Cultural & Creative Series present how the center works and what have been achieved. It's quite exciting to see such great accomplishments that the center has been got in Chinese cultural communication and talent cultivation.

Accompanied by the accelerated globalization, technology innovation capacity and cultural communication capacity have grown into the core competence in the international arena. The popularity of Hollywood blockbuster and iPhone exemplifies the great power boasted from the converging advanced technology and popular culture. Upgraded from an economic giant to an economic power, it's necessary for China to undergo the change from "Made in China" to "Created in China", and that's why technological innovation should go hand in hand with cultural communication.

Since the extensive and profound Chinese culture breeds rich creativity, many abstract images derive from myth, philosophy and poem, while some concrete ones come from such traditional Chinese images as plum, orchid, bamboo, chrysanthemum, pavilion, etc. The innovative development of Chinese culture requires the in-depth fusion of humanity, arts and technology. The inner meaning of upgrading China from a manufacturer of quantity to one of quality is embodied in the products that both represent the modern technology and satisfy our living and aesthetic needs.

Nowadays, the economic and consumption structures have been upgraded rapidly, as the result of which, the demand for differentiated and individualized products is growing. If we can soften the powerful productivity of China by using smart technology, make the creative ideas coming from multi-culture blend into individualized design and customized service, fuel the product design and manufacturing with the technology, arts and humanity, it would be more possible to fulfill China's move from "Made in China" to "Created in China", also to make greater contribution to global economy and human civilization.

The core of mass entrepreneurship and innovation is to show our respect for everyone's right of starting their own businesses and making innovations and to tap their potentials. The motive of such an encouragement is to make more people "being enabled", which means that the latest achievements of technological development can be applied to more entrepreneurship and innovation cases. In this way, the traditional elements of Chinese culture can enlighten more creators proceeding from arts, aesthetics and experience to design products satisfying diversified needs. This is the right way to invigorate mass entrepreneurship and innovation.

WAN Gang
CPPCC Vice Chairman and Former Minister of Science & Technology

自序

"艺术与心灵成长"是我长期以来在同济大学开设的一门通识课。授课过程中，我结合自身的艺术教育背景和心灵静修旅程，与年轻的学生们一起探讨如何从充满爱与美的艺术世界中得到启迪，获得心灵成长。机缘成熟时，我编辑了这本彩色印刷的文选，望与更多的读者进行心灵交流。

我们为什么需要艺术？

我们需要艺术，因为它能够赋予我们爱与美的享受。在人类活动的数万年历史中形成了不同的文明、丰富的思想、卓越的发现和发明。艺术也是人类文明的产物，艺术与人类共生共存，相互影响。专注思考一个艺术作品，听一首音乐，看一部电影，我们的心灵会得到某种慰藉和舒心之感。

我们需要艺术，因为它是人类文明和知识的载体。艺术形式的人文属性把我们与绵延数千年的历史联系在一起，让我们通过艺术来了解历史，从中获得有益的教育和启迪，使我们的生活有了意义。

我们需要艺术，因为它能够引发人类的共鸣。艺术家用他独立思考的能力和跳出群体思维模式的勇气为观众提供了延伸经历的新鲜见解，让欣赏者从中获得情感与观念上的认同。艺术的背后，是生命的思考与绽放。

我们需要艺术，因为它是世界通用的。这种非语言的交流没有沟通障碍，它有助于情感的表达与理解。任何一件艺术作品都可以雕琢我们的灵魂。

我们为什么要心灵成长？

心灵成长是为了能让心灵不断找回自己本来的力量。在人类文明的发展中，我们运用科学认识外部世界，而通过表达来审视自己的精神世界。我们不仅是物质的存在，也是精神的存在，生活不仅是为了追逐物质满足，更是为了实现自我的精神价值。正如鸟儿有两个翅膀才能飞翔一样，人类也需要精神和物质两方面的平衡，才能拥有自然、和谐的生活。

心灵成长就是接受自己，爱自己。生活中不会一直充满绚烂的瞬间，更多的是趋于平凡的经历。每个人的生命里都有接踵而来的难题，既没有必要艳羡别人的精彩人生，也没有必要因为自己的无能为力而妄自菲薄。拼尽全力，做自己喜欢的事，成为真正的自己。每个个体都是独一无二的存在，每一场经历都是独属于自己的故事。

心灵成长就是放下执念和过多的欲望。人生的痛苦往往来源于过多的欲望，其中大部分的欲望是没有必要的。只要让未被察觉的思维控制着你的生活，痛苦就会随之自然而然地产生。如埃克哈特·托利在《当下的力量》一书中所说："如果你正在做的事情中没有喜悦、自在和轻松，这并不意味着你需要改变你正在做的事情，而是需要改变你做事的方式。"只有放下执念，关注当下，才能轻松前行。

希望艺术与心灵成长能帮助我们激发和尝试驾驭生命能量的洪流，让我们能够优雅地处理生活中大大小小的事情，给自己的生活带来更多的张力和迸发的潜力。这种生活就像是康定斯基的作品一样，看似是几何形状的叠加，多种色调的碰撞，或混乱，或明快，但点线面之间的关系和丰富的颜色运用构成了充满逻辑与动感的画面，他的作品拥有与心灵节拍相吻合的节奏……

漫漫历史，大千世界，人们生活各异，但艺术给予人的力量永存。当我们学会体验和欣赏艺术，艺术传达的不仅仅是一种令人赏心悦目的美感，也隐含了对生命的热爱和对时代的思考，将会赋予我们的心灵更多的启发与滋养。让我们一起：

学会发现生活中的美好事物，并心存感激；

学会关注当下，用不抱怨的状态面对生活中的挫折；

学会在繁忙的工作学习中让自己放松；

学会以健康的生活方式爱自己；

还有更多的成长值得我们去探讨……

最后，老子言："上善若水，水善利万物而不争，处众人之所恶，故几于道。"愿所有读者能若水一般，清静柔和，至善至纯。

俞　鹰

Editor's Preface

Art and Spiritual Growth is a general course that I have offered at Tongji University for many years. In this course, I combine my art education background and meditation journey to discuss with young students how to get enlightenment from the art world that is full of love and beauty, and obtain spiritual growth. When it was time, I edited this color-printed anthology, hoping to communicate with more readers.

Why do we need art?

We need art because it can give us the enjoyment of love and beauty. In the long history of mankind, different civilizations, rich ideas, outstanding discoveries and inventions have been formed. Art is also a product of human civilization. Art and mankind coexist and influence each other. By thinking over a work of art, listening to a piece of music, watching a movie, our heart will get a certain sense of comfort and consolation.

We need art because it is the carrier of human civilization. The humanistic nature of the art forms connects us with thousands of years of history, allowing us to understand history through art, obtain knowledge and enlightenment from it, and make our lives meaningful.

We need art because it can resonate with human beings. Artists have the courage to break out of group thinking. They think independently and provide us with fresh insights that extend our experience, allowing us to gain emotional and conceptual recognition. Behind art there is the philosophy and bloom of life.

We need art because it is universal. This kind of nonverbal communication has no barriers. Art helps express and understand emotions. Any work of art can carve our spirit.

Why do we need spiritual growth?

The purpose of spiritual growth is to allow our mind to constantly regain its original strength. In the development of human civilization, we understand the external world by learning science and examine our own spiritual world through expression. We are not only a material existence but also a spiritual one. Life is not only for the pursuit of material satisfaction but also for the realization of our spiritual value. Just as a bird has two wings to fly, humans also need a balance of spiritual and material aspects, so as to live a natural and harmonious life.

Spiritual growth is to accept and love yourself. Life will not always be full of splendid moments, but more ordinary experiences. Everyone will encounter numerous problems. There is no need to envy others, and there is no need to humiliate oneself because of one's inability. Do your best, do what you like, and become who you are! Each individual is unique, and every experience is an inimitable story.

Spiritual growth is to let go of obsessions and excessive desires. The pain of life often comes from excessive desires, most of which are unnecessary. As long as you let undetected thoughts control your life, the pain will follow naturally. As Eckhart Tolle put it in his book *The Power of Now*: "If there is no joy, ease, or lightness in what you are doing, it does not necessarily mean that you need to change what you are doing. It may be sufficient to change the how. How is always more important than what." Only by letting go of obsessions and paying more attention to the present can you move forward easily.

I hope that Art and Spiritual Growth can inspire people to float on the stream of life, so that we can gracefully handle everything, and bring more flexibility and potential to life. This kind of life is just like Wassily Kandinsky's artwork. At first sight, there is a superposition of geometric shapes, a contrast of multiple tones, with lights and shadows. But the connection between dots, lines and surfaces and the rich use of colors constitute a dynamic appearance. His works always have a rhythm that matches people's mind...

With a splendid history and a vast world, people now live in different ways. But the power that art gives people will last forever. When we learn to appreciate art, art conveys not only a pleasing sense of beauty, but also implies love for life and thinking about the times, which will give us more inspiration and nourishment. Let us be together:

Learn to discover beauty in life and be grateful;
Learn to pay attention to the present and face the setbacks in life without complaining;
Learn to relax in the busy schedule of working and learning;
Learn to love yourself with a healthy lifestyle;
There is more to explore...

To sum up, as the ancient Chinese philosopher Lao Tzu said: "A person with superior goodness is like water. Water is good in benefiting all beings. Without contending with any. Situated in places shunned by many others. Thereby it is near Tao." May all the readers be like water, quiet, soft, perfect and pure.

YU Ying

目录

前言
宁静与健康
Serenity and Health

顺其自然，最好的办法就是保持健康。人的身体每天都会自动代谢一定比例的细胞。如果你保持乐观，身体就会释放些特殊物质，通过血液流遍全身，促进细胞的生长和再生。宁静而快乐的心态看似无为，但它发送出的信号却能让身体无不为。运动就像在和身体一起思考，而不是被动地从大脑接收信号，特别是像游泳、太极和瑜伽等无竞争性的运动，会向大脑发送健康的信号。我们为运动而生，而情感强化了我们的身体系统。运动激发了身体的信号系统，让大脑保持冷静，不要烦躁。然后，大脑向细胞发出"前进"的信号，推进细胞新陈代谢。因此，健康的身体基于健康的心理，健康的心理又源于健康的身体。它们一起创造了无为和无不为之间一种健康的平衡。所以某种程度上，你的心理决定了你的细胞健康与否。

在我看来，乐观的信息会告诉细胞："活着是有价值的，身体需要健康的细胞。"而消极的信息会告诉细胞："没有必要再产生新细胞，而且现有的细胞也会衰退老化。"压力源于克制某种冲动。在过去，当生命安全受到威胁时，从心理上，人们不允许自己什么都不做，所以做出一定的反抗；在现代社会里，就是你的钱财或社会地位受到威胁时，也尽量克制着想反抗的冲动，从而出现了压力。长期的压力、担心或悔恨会不断产生一些化学物质，导致你的细胞为了应付短暂的冲动而忽略了长期的健康，让你觉得细胞随着时间推移不断老化。抑郁会危害生命，自杀只是一方面，另一方面还会因为担忧而毁坏细胞。我认为，大多数自杀者还没有从生理上结束生命之前，就已经从心理上终结了自己。不健康的心理能缓慢地从潜意识上终结生命。不过，我们可以拯救这种慢性死亡。

为了健康，你必须遵循自然法则，找到更好的生活方式并从假想的种种责任中把自己解放出来。对自己好一点，如果你不知道该做什么，就什么都不做，这并不是犯罪。就像一幅典型的中国画《渔夫图》，渔夫或满载而归，或空手而归，但他的心是平静而健康的，因为他完成了一天的工作。他现在无事可做，就任涟漪轻推小船，清风拂过脸颊，见夕阳西下。

大自然是伟大的治愈者，带着好奇观察大自然，你会发现大自然才是无限的，静静地做深呼吸，让自己沉浸于这美好的无限中吧；用谦卑欣赏的眼神凝视它，从非自然状态中释放自己吧。告诉自然"我相信你"，它也会回报给你惊喜。让自然拥抱你，它会驱走你不健康的心理，使你拥有平静的内心和充满活力的身体。

——摘自赵启光，《无为无不为》

The best way to let nature follow its course is to be healthy. Every day, you replace a certain percentage of your cells. When you are optimistic, your body releases specific substances that move through your blood, telling your cells to grow and reproduce. A serene and merry mind seems to do nothing, but it sends out signals telling the cells to do everything. Exercise is like thinking with the body. Instead of receiving signals from the mind, exercises especially noncompetitive exercises like swimming, Tai Chi, and Yoga - make your body send back healthy signals to the mind.

We are built to move, and emotion reinforces our system. Exercise triggers the signaling system that tells our mind to be calm, to stop agonizing. As a result, the mind sends "go ahead" signals to cells for the daily processes of cell replacement. Thus, the sound mind builds on a sound body, and the sound body on a sound mind. Together, they create a healthy balance of doing nothing and doing everything. So to a certain extent, your mind decides whether your cells will be healthy.

As I see it, good signals tell your cells that living is worthwhile, and healthy cells are in demand; bad signals

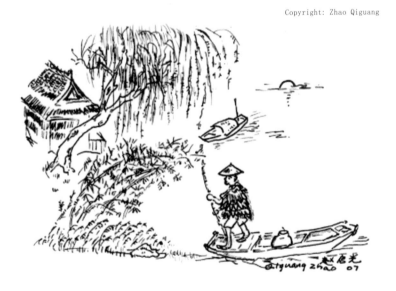

A day's work is done, a fisherman returns to his cottage behind the willow trees.

tell your cells that reproduction is not necessary, and the existing cells can decay. Stress is the suppressed intention to act, the mentality of not allowing yourself to do nothing in the face of dangers that threatened your physical security in the past or your financial or social safety now. Long-term stress, worry, and regret produce a steady trickle of chemicals that cause your cells to neglect their long-term health to keep you wired for short-term action, in effect telling your cells to decay overtime. Depression threatens your life not only through suicide but also with the cell-damaging effects of worrying. Most suicidal people do not physically commit suicide, but a suicidal mentality can terminate the body just as effectively. The mind can kill the body slowly and subconsciously. This slow dying can be reversed.

To be healthy, follow the course of nature, find a better way of living, and liberate yourself from the chains of imagined responsibility. Be generous with yourself. It is not a crime to do nothing when you do not know what to do. A typical theme in traditional Chinese painting is the fisherman returning home. His boat may be full or empty, but he is serene and healthy because he has done his day's work, and he will have nothing to do now, except let the ripple touch his boat, the breeze caress his face, and the sun set.

Nature is the great healer. Stare at it with curious eyes and know your limitations; breathe it with an empty belly, and immerse yourself in limitlessness, contemplate it with humble appreciation, and liberate yourself from unnatural bonds. Tell nature, "I trust you," and nature will not fail to give you surprises. Allow nature to embrace you, and nature will take your unhealthy mentality away and return you a calm mind and a rejuvenated body.

From ZHAO Qiguang, *Do Noting and Do Everything*

意识的进化：三体
The Evolution of Consciousness Series
The Three Bodies

本篇是葛木雷什·D.巴特尔所写的关于意识进化的系列文章的第一部分，关于灵性修习如何设计，用以帮助意识的扩展和进化。

当谈论为自己编织命运和未来的时候，我们的意思是什么？世俗意义上来说，我们都想过上好日子。从一间卧室的公寓，想换成五间卧室的房子；从一家工厂发展到拥有十家工厂；我想从普通职员晋升为CEO；还想有个幸福美满的家庭，并且孩子们长大以后也有富足的生活。

从灵性的视角来看，我们关心的是更加远大的景象。为了更深入地探索，我们首先要描述一下人类的构造。我们有个物理上的身体，有血有肉，这是最为固有的部分。尽管会有一点变化，根据我们的生活方式，身体不会有很大变化。身体的进化需要比一个生世更为久远的时间，所以我们不能期望身体在此生就能进化。身体与物质相关。

我们还有细体，也被称为灵体或精神体，它与能量和振动相关。这也就是我们所说的心和智。

我们的第三个身体是因果体，是我们存在的原因，也被称作灵魂。因果体与绝对的虚无之境有关，是存在的基础。因果体是纯净的、不变的以及永恒的，因此它不需要进化。

对于身体和因果体，我们不可能期望其进化。当我们想要改变自己的思维或行为模式的时候，在任何自我提升的过程中，不论是心理上的或是精神上的，能够改变或者进化的是中间层——细体。灵性命运与细体的净化密切相关，通过去除包裹着细体的那些面纱。

在矿物界，三体连接如此紧密以致很难分开；它们没有太多自由。在某种程度上，它们可以自由振动，于是它们就有了不同的特质，而人们就将其命名为金、铝、铌，等等。

在植物界，三体稍微松散一点。你去看一棵树，你如何知道它有细体在回应？你是否看到过花朵在日出的时候绽放？花朵如何知道呢？它们如此确切地做出反应，根据太阳的移动而转动。有一种叫作含羞草的植物，当你触碰它的时候叶子就会卷拢。当微风吹过或是有暴风的时候，树的枝叶随风舞动，但是当有人想要折断树枝的时候，这棵树会变得不安。你可以感受得到。植物的细体和因果体紧紧相连，细体没有太多的表现。

在动物身上有着更大的分隔距离，而在人类身上，三体是容易分开的或者连接很松散，在不同的人身上，分离的程度也不尽相同。吠陀哲学中所说的三种特性——悦性、惰性和激性——取决于三体的连接程度是松散还是牢固。

一个悦性的人，其细体可以随意移动，而一个惰性的人就像一块石头一样。有的人可以决胜于千里之外，而有的人由于脑力有限，甚至很难知道周围发生的事情。即使你告诉他们，其思维也很难理解。有时，当我们交流的时候，有些概念对其他人来说非常费解，因为那些人的细体无法理解。

所以在细体的层面上，我们可以选择进化；超越动物层面的存在达到人的层面, 甚至达到神圣的层面, 通过扩展我们意识的范围而达到。

我们如何描绘细体, 而细体又是如何进化的呢? 细体有四个主要的功能值得我们思考:

意 (chit) (Chit or consciousness)

思 (manas) (Manas or our contemplative faculty)

智 (buddhi) (Buddhi or intellect)

自我 (ahankar) (Ahankar or ego)

这四种功能在我们的进化中都有自身的作用, 在下文中, 我们将进一步探讨。

This is the first in a series of articles by Kamlesh D. Patel about the evolution of consciousness, and how spiritual practices are designed to help consciousness expand and evolve.

When we talk about weaving a destiny, a future for ourselves, what do we mean? In the worldly sense, we want a good life. From my one-bedroom apartment, I want a five-bedroom house; from owning one factory I hope to own ten factories; I dream of being promoted from the position of a clerk to that of a CEO; I want a happy and fulfilling family life, and to raise children who also have fulfilling lives.

From the spiritual perspective, we are concerned with a much bigger picture. In order to explore this further, we need to first describe the human make up. We have a physical body, made of flesh and blood that is the most solid part of us. While it changes a little bit, according to how we live our lives, it doesn't change much. Physical evolution happens over longer periods than one lifetime, so we don't expect our physical body to evolve in this life. The physical body to evolve in this life. The physical body is associated with matter.

We also have a subtle body, also known as the astral or mental body, that is associated with energy and vibration. This is what we call the heart and mind.

The third body we have is our causal body, the cause of our existence, which is also known as the soul. The causal body is associated with the absolute state of nothingness, the substratum of existence. This causal body is pure, unchanging and immutable, so it is does not need to evolve.

With the physical and the causal bodies, we cannot expect to find evolutionary changes. When we want to change our thinking and our patterns of behaviour, during any process of self-development, be it psychological or spiritual, what evolves or transforms is the middle layer, the subtle body. Spiritual destiny has everything to do with the purification of the subtle body by removing the layers that surround it.

In the mineral kingdom, all three bodies are so closely tied together that it is difficult to separate them; they don't have much freedom. To the extent to which they can free themselves vibrationally, they have different qualities and we give them names like Gold, Lead, Osmium, etc.

In the plant kingdom, the three bodies are a little looser. Look at a tree. How do you know it has a subtle body that responds? Have you seen flowers that open up when the sun comes? How do they know? They respond so nicely, turning as the sun moves. There is also a plant called Lajvanti, and when you touch it the leaves fold in. When there is a breeze, or even a storm, the leaves and branches of trees dance, but the moment someone tries to cut the branch of a tree, it becomes agitated. You can feel it. In plants, the subtle body and the causal body are very tightly tied together, and the subtle body cannot express much.

In animals, there is a still greater separation, and in human beings all the three bodies are labile or loosely connected. Among different human beings, there are also differences in separation. The three gunas in vedic philosophy – tamasic, rajasic and sattvik – are based on how loosely or how strongly the bodies are connected.

In a sattvik person, the subtle body can move around, whereas a tamasic person is more stone-like. One person can think of something somewhere else, but another person with limited mental capacity may not grasp what is happening around them. Even if you tell them about it, their mind cannot reach there. Sometimes, when we communicate, certain concepts are not understood by the other person because of the subtle body's inability to grasp them.

So at the level of the subtle body, we can choose to evolve and go beyond the animal level of existence to the human level to the divine level, by expanding our field of consciousness.

How can we describe the subtle body, and how does it evolve? There are four main functions of the subtle body that we will consider and they are:

Chit or consciousness,

Manas or our contemplative faculty,

Buddhi or intellect, and

Ahankar or ego.

They all have a role to play in our evolution, and in the next article of the series we will explore them further.

意识的进化：细体

The Evolution of Consciousness Series
The Subtle Body

在上文中，葛木雷什·D. 巴特尔描述了三种主要的机体，它们在一起形成了地球生物的基础。在本文中，他将深度探索三体其中之一的细体， 以及它如何进化。

哪一体在进化?

理解了我们有三体——身体、细体、因果体——我们会问是哪一体在进化?

灵魂是不可改变的，它是纯洁的、绝对的以及固定不变的，因此因果体不会进化。

身体也不会改变太多。其结构是固定的，尽管在体重、姿态及身材等方面可能会有一些较小的变化，但我们在此生却无法长出更多手臂，或者可以飞翔的翅膀，或者尾巴。

能够进化的是细体，因此可以设定我们的未来。细体的变化在于我们对其净化和简化的程度，灵魂的愉悦因此发光并从内在散发出来，由此，我们可以发现意识的进化。

细体

细体是振动的区域，也是心脑区域。根据我们如何管理这个区域，这里既可以充满混乱与嘈杂，就如风暴中咆哮的海洋，或者是另一极端，水平如镜，即便一根羽毛也能引起涟漪。在这里，灵性修习有着重要的作用，因为它为我们提供了方法去调整、净化及简化这个区域，带来纯净、安宁与平和。

在瑜伽哲学中，心被认为是思维的活动之地。这是一个非常大的话题。现在让我们来探索其中的意义。

在这个振动的区域中，细体有四种主要的功能——意识（chit），心思（manas），智力（buddhi），自我（ahankar）。它们以一种相互作用的方式一起工作，形成了我们所说的思维。

在这四种功能中，意识是我们关注的焦点。另外三种也存在于意识之中。意识无异于画家的画布，其他三种功能每日在意识之中协奏。

我们如何主动地让意识扩展和进化？仅仅希望如此是不够的。我们需要明白心灵修习如何通过创造一种状态让思维逐渐在越来越深的层面上安静，并打开内在的宇宙，从而有助进化。

照片：那泽民摄

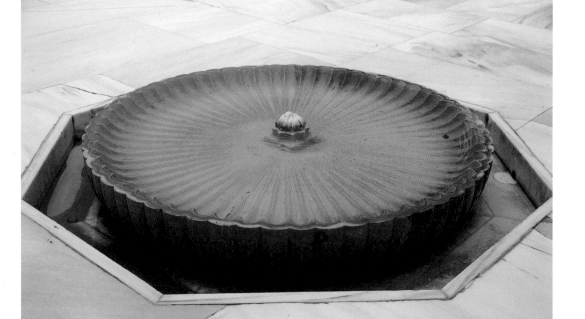

在身体的层面，如果想让身体的肌肉变得更强壮，那就需要去锻炼身体。同样，为了让头脑能够进化，从而让意识能够扩展，就必须运用生命存在的精细层面。首先，重要的一点是需要知道，意识的进化与获取知识无关。其次，没有智力、心思和自我这三种细体的帮助让意识摆脱束缚，意识本身并不会扩展和进化。智力必须进化，以帮助意识进行扩展；自我也必须进化，有助于意识的进化。

冥想

冥想在这个过程中有什么作用呢？我们通过冥想来陶冶头脑，无序的头脑会受到欲望、渴求、恐惧和习惯的驱使，有很多不同的方向。由于分散到不同的渠道，大脑会变弱。相反，有序的头脑会带来专注，并能提升安康。除非并且直至我们正确地冥想，以及正确地陶冶头脑，否则我们的意识不会进化。

通过冥想，智力、心思和自我都会得到精炼和改善。尤其是心思，当学会简化我们的思想过程从多渠道转化为单一渠道的时候，便能让其深入感觉。这样慢慢地会从"思考"中培养出"感觉"的习惯。

进一步发展冥想的状态

在一天之中保持和培养在冥想中所获得的状态，这是一次良好冥想所带来的副产品，能够帮助我们陶冶及深化头脑甚至达到更高层次。当处于这种持续的觉知或思念的内在状态的时候，我们便不会让自己的画布被破坏，所以能够保持清醒。画布会一直保持干净，并且不会被我

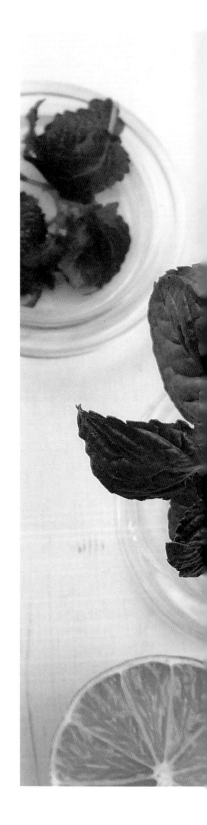

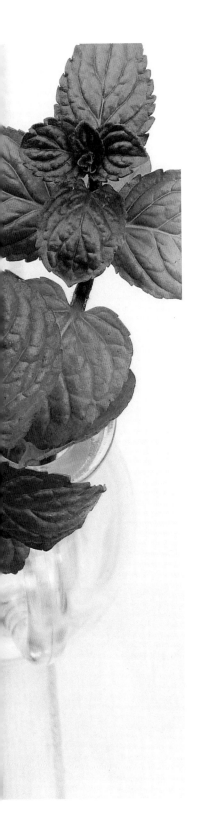

们形成的各种各样的印记所破坏。

想象一下，心脑振动区域中有一个意识谱，涵盖了潜意识、意识和超意识的状态。印度近代哲学家、印度教改革家辨喜大师曾说过，"意识只不过是潜意识与超意识两个大洋间的一层薄膜"。或者可以想象潜意识是一个大海，意识就像陆地的表面，而超意识就像通向宇宙的天空。随着我们的进化，我们的意识同时扩展至潜意识与超意识的领域之中，遨游于人类潜能的宽广无限之中。另一种说法是，从表面开始，我们会越来越深入内心的浩瀚之中。

智力与祈愿

在这个深入的过程中，智力会越来越变得以心为基础。直觉与灵感得到发展，而智力得到了很好的调节，就像是敏感的天线能捕捉到心的信号。智力进化到智慧的状态。我们常常认为有智慧的人会做出明智的决定，但是在这里我们会走得更远，进入一个不同的维度，我们不再需要选择，因为心的智慧是纯洁和正确的。

有知识的人和有智慧的人之间有着很大的差别，在这里灵性修习的祈愿能帮助我们从只有知识到拥有智慧。祈愿会让我们回到内心，与本源相连，我们能够放下过去所犯的错误，并下决心不再犯同样的错误。这难道不是智慧吗？反之，如果我们听任自己日复一日、持续不停地犯着愚蠢的错误，我们便没有智慧。当我们从心底希望能够获得改变并寻求帮助的时候，就会变得有智慧。当我们每时每刻都处在这样的态度之中时，智慧便会盛放。

智慧在于将感官付诸最佳用途。智慧是以最小的投入获得最大的产出。用最小的行为我们就能获得最大的成果。只有冥想状态的头脑，只有在我们的日常生活中通过冥想状态下的言行，才有可能期盼如此美好的成果。

通过清心净化及简化细体

为了实现这一点，心脑区域必须得到净化，否则就像奢望透过污浊动荡的湖水见到湖底一样，终不可得。奔腾的头脑不会清净。因此，清除过去印记的灵性修习对于意识进化来说就十分必要。

自我

细体的第三个方面就是自我。无论意识的扩展或进化是否能够发生，自我都起着非常关键的作用。在所有的传统中，自我经常都被灵性修行者当作坏人，可是自我也是我们进化的基础。它是思维的活跃功能——做和想的功能——在日常生活的每一方面我们都需要它，甚至是渴求进化。它给予我们身份。它是一种活跃或原初的力量。如果能够智慧地使用它，它就会很好地为我们服务，就像其他资源一样，但它经常被滥用，而这就是我们通常所说的自我中心。当自我被应用于自私的目的时，我们就会变得自负和自大，相反，假如我们不断地精炼自我，意识将会得到快速进化。

精炼自我是什么意思？我们越是谦卑，自私的增长就越少。所有伟大的灵性老师都非常重视性格的塑造这个方面。他们是如此推崇这一品质，无论付出什么代价都要保持谦卑，无论是对待一个小孩、一个穷人，还是一个陌生

照片：王锐光摄

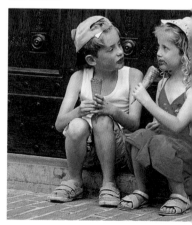

人。这里面的哲学是,认为自己很了不起,并没有什么不对,但总是要认为面前的人比自己更伟大。

自我就像是黑洞,会对我们的意识造成强大的吸引力。它不允许意识扩展。正如地球引力不允许我们进入无限的太空一样,自我也能将意识束缚于其核心之中。例如,一个非常自恋的人处于退化的过程,意识缩小到自己的核心,可能会变得像一块石头。相反,通过精炼自我从而超越与自我之间的关系,变得越来越谦卑,意识将扩展至无限。

自我会以很多方式显现。例如,在一场音乐会中,当我作为一名乐手欢乐地吹奏长笛的时候,就会释放出许多快乐,而听众也会有所回应。但作为一名艺术家,除非我能经常超越之前的表演,否则不会高兴。这时显现出来的自我让我能表演出色。但如果想着没有人能比我演奏得更好,这就是不受欢迎的自我显现了。自我能够成为我们的好朋友,帮助我们超越之前的纪录。

心思

细体的第四个功能就是心思,其功能是沉思。在冥想的过程中,第一步就是将我们心中大量繁杂的念头变为一个念头,例如在满心冥想之中,这个念头就是心中神圣的光之源。但是在整个冥想的过程中,没必要一直想着这个念头。在某个时刻这个念头应离开,以便让思想的对象可以在心中感觉到。

如果你在整个冥想的过程中都在想着这个念头,你会感到头痛,而意识也不会扩展。这个最初的念头只是一个跳板,让我们能够更加深入,这样才能融化于圣光显现的感觉之中。你应当去感觉那种显现,而当你去感觉的时候,慢慢地你会消失,甚至连感觉也没有了。自我消失了,你甚至都不在那里体验了。

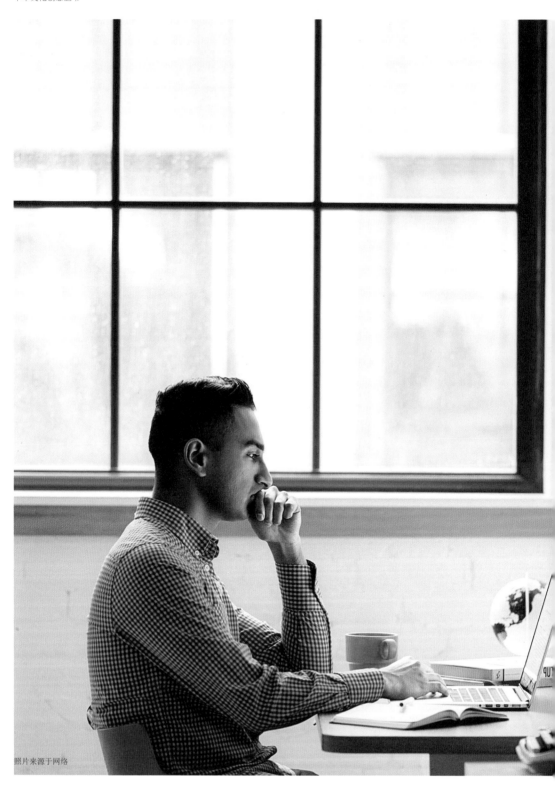

照片来源于网络

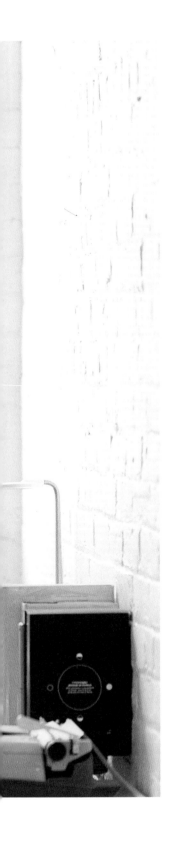

所以，当心思通过冥想修习进化时，感觉会增强，最终，我们超越了感觉到达存在的状态，然后进入成为的状态，最后不再成为，而是融入了存在的绝对状态。

意识

所以，智力、心思和自我通过灵性修习而进化，由此细体会变得更加轻盈、更加纯洁和更加简单，如同只有细微涟漪的平静湖面。如此意识便能得到扩展和进化。

我们要以自己得到的已经扩展的意识来做什么? 假设我有某种特定的思维状态，我意识到这种状态非常好。冥想之后我会去工作，仅仅是保持那种状态是不够的;我必须能够主动地、有意识地去辐射出那种状态，带着这样的信心——无论走到哪里，都将散发出它的芬芳。

所以，在冥想之后要思考一阵，"我内在的状态也存在于我的外在。我周围的一切都沉浸于同样的状态之中。当我看着别人、与他们交谈或聆听他们，或者我处于安静之中时，就让这种状态传遍周围"。让意识扩展到能到达的任何地方。

In the first article of the series, "The Three Bodies", Kamlesh D. Patel described the three main bodies that together form the base of life forms on earth. In this second article, he explores one of these in depth, the subtle body, and how it evolves.

Which body evolves?

Understanding that we have these three bodies – physical, subtle and causal – we can then ask, which of these bodies is evolving?

The soul is immutable. It is pure, absolute and unchangeable, and so the causal body does not evolve.

The physical body cannot change much. Its structure is fixed, although some minor changes can occur in weight, posture and fitness etc., but we cannot grow extra arms, wings to fly or a tail in this lifetime.

It is the subtle body that can evolve, so that we can design our destiny. It changes according to how we purify and simplify it, so that the joy of the soul shines and radiates from within, and through this process we find the evolution of consciousness.

The Subtle Body

The subtle body is a vibrational field; the heart-mind field. Depending on how we manage this field, it can either be turbulent and complex, like a roaring ocean during a storm, or, at the other extreme, it can be like a still pond where even a feather landing on the surface creates ripples. This is where a spiritual practice has a vital role to play, as it gives us the techniques to regulate, purify and simplify this field, bringing clarity, stillness and peace.

In yogic philosophy the heart is known as the field of action for the mind. This is a vast topic. Let's start to explore what this means.

There are four main functions of the subtle body within

this vibrational field – consciousness (*chit*), thinking and feeling (*manas*), intellect (*buddhi*) and ego (*ahankar*). They work in an interactive way together to make up what we know as the mind.

Of these four, consciousness is our focus here. The other three have their existence in consciousness. Consciousness is as good as a canvas to a painter, and within consciousness the play of the other three bodies is orchestrated daily.

How do we actively allow our consciousness to expand and evolve? It is not enough just to wish it so. We need to understand how a spiritual practice contributes towards this evolution by creating the conditions for stilling the mind progressively at deeper and deeper levels, and opening up the inner universe.

At a physical level, when I want to strengthen my body mus-cles I have to exercise my body. Similarly, for

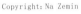

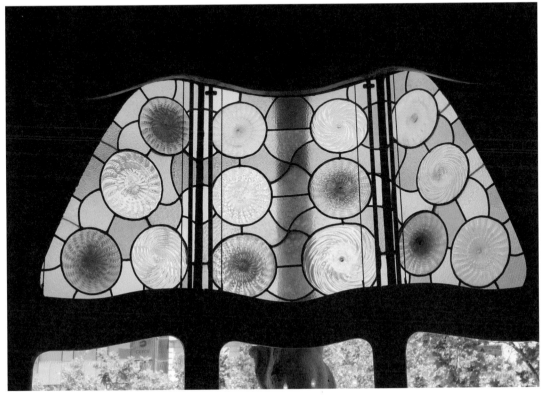

the mind to evolve so that consciousness can expand, I must use what belongs to that subtle plane of existence. First, it is important to understand that the evolution of consciousness has nothing to do with the acquisition of knowledge. Second, consciousness in itself will not expand or evolve without the help of *buddhi, manas* and *ahankar* to free it. Intellect has to evolve to help expand consciousness and ego must evolve, contributing to the evolution of consciousness.

Meditation

What does meditation have to do with this? We meditate to regulate our minds. An unregulated mind is pulled by wishes and desires, fears and habits, in many different directions. The mind becomes weak as it scatters in many different channels. In contrast, a regulated mind brings focus, and promotes well-being. Unless and until we meditate properly, and unless and until we regulate our minds properly, our consciousness will not evolve.

Manas, buddhi and *ahankar* are all refined and developed through meditation, especially *manas* as we learn to simplify our thinking process from many channels to one channel, then deepen it to feeling. Thus the habit of "feeling" is slowly cultivated from "thinking".

Developing the Meditative State Further

Holding and nurturing the condition received in meditation throughout the day is a byproduct of good meditation, and helps us regulate and deepen the mind to an even higher level. When we are in this state of constant awareness or remem-brance of the inner state, we do not allow our canvas to be spoilt, so consciousness remains afresh. The canvas remains clean and is not destroyed by the multifarious impressions we form.

Imagine the heart-mind vibrational field having a spectrum of consciousness spanning the subconscious, conscious and superconscious states. Swami Vivekananda once said, "Con-sciousness is a mere film between two oceans, the subcon-scious and the superconscious." Or you can imagine the subconscious as being like the ocean, consciousness like the surface of the land, and superconsciousness like the sky going out into the universe. As we evolve, our consciousness expands into both the subconscious and superconscious realms, travelling through the vast infinity of the human potential. Another way of saying this is that we go deeper and deeper into the vastness of the heart, from our starting point at the surface.

Buddhi and Prayer

In this process of diving deeper, the intellect, buddhi, becomes more and more heart-based. Intuition and inspiration develop, and buddhi becomes fine-tuned, like a sensitive antenna picking up the signals of the heart. Intellect evolves into a state of wisdom. Often we think of a wise person as someone who makes wise choices, but here we go further into a different dimension where choice is no longer required, as the heart's wisdom is pure and correct.

There is a big difference between an intellectual person and a wise person, and here the spiritual practice of prayer helps us to move from mere intellect to wisdom. Prayer

Copyright: Wang Ruiguang

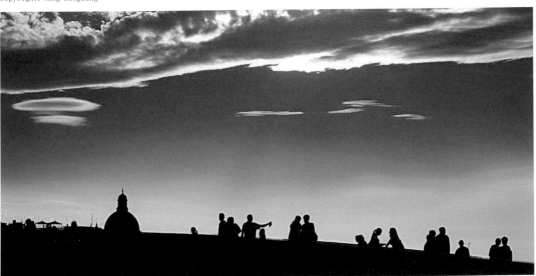

takes us into the heart, connecting us to the Source, where we are able to let go of any mistakes we have made, deciding not to make the same mistakes again. Is this not wisdom? Whereas if we succumb to making foolish mistakes day after day, hour after hour, we are not becoming wiser. We become wiser when we wish to change from the bottom of our hearts and ask for help to do so. When we live with this attitude every moment, wisdom flourishes.

Wisdom is to utilise all our faculties at their best. Wisdom is to have the maximum output with the minimum input. With minimum action we have the maximum result. Only with a meditative mind, only through meditative acts in our day-to-day life, can we expect to have such good results.

Purifying and Simplifying the Subtle Body Through Cleaning

For this to happen, the heart-mind field has to be purified, otherwise it is like expecting to see the bottom of a lake through muddy, turbulent water. There is no clarity in a turbulent mind. The spiritual practice of cleaning past impressions is therefore also necessary for consciousness to evolve.

Copyright: Wang Ruiguang

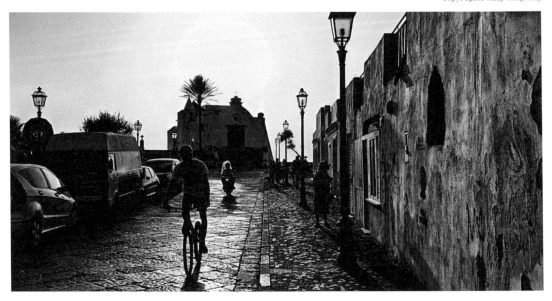

Ahankar

The third aspect of the subtle body is ego, *ahankar*. Ego plays a vital role in whether or not expansion or evolution of consciousness occurs. Ego is often seen as the bad guy by spiritual practitioners of all traditions, but ego is also essential for our evolution. It is the active function of the mind – the doing, thinking function – and we need it in every apect of daily life, even to have the craving to evolve. It gives us our identity. It is the activating or initiating force. If it is used wisely, it serves us well, like any other resource, but it is often misused, and this is what we commonly refer to as being egotistical. When ego is used for selfish purpose, we become arrogant and self-important, whereas if we constantly refine the ego, consciousness develops very rapidly.

What does it mean to refine the ego? The more humility we have, the less the egotistical proliferations. All great spiritual teachers have given so much importance to this aspect of character formation. They have valued this quality so highly that humility at any cost must be maintained, whether towards a child, a poor person or a stranger. The philosophy here is that there is nothing wrong in thinking yourself to be great, but always think the other person in front of you is greater.

Ego can be like a black hole. It can have the greatest gravi-tational pull upon our consciousness. It will not allow consciousness to expand. Just as the earth's gravitational pull does not allow us to fall into infinite space, likewise our ego can hold consciousness to its core. An example of this is a very narcissistic person, who is undergoing a devolutionary process where consciousness contracts in on itself to its core, and can become like a stone. In contrast, by transcending the relationship with the ego by refining it, becoming more and more humble, consciousness can expand infinitely.

Ego manifests in many ways. For example, in a music concert, when I am happily playing my flute as a performer, it gives so much joy and the audience reciprocates accordingly. But as an artist, I will not be happy unless I surpass my previous performances all the time. The manifested ego makes me perform well. But to think that no one can play the flute better than myself is not a welcome manifestation of ego. Ego can be our best friend in helping us outperform our own past records.

Manas

The fourth function of the subtle body is manas, which is the function of contemplation. During meditation, the first step is to bring the mind from many and varied thoughts to one thought, for example in Heartfulness it is the source of Divine

Light in the heart. But it is not necessary that all throughout the meditation this thought should haunt us. The thought should leave at some point so that the object of thought can be felt in the heart.

If all you do is think this one thought throughout the medi-tation, you will have a headache and consciousness will not expand. This initial thought is just the springboard, to take us deeper so that we dissolve in the feeling of the presence of the Divine Light. You have to feel that presence and while you are feeling that presence slowly you disappear, and even feeling is gone. The ego is gone; you are not even there to experience it.

So as *manas* evolves through a meditation practice, feeling develops, and eventually we go beyond feeling to a state of being, then to a state of becoming, and finally unbecoming to merge into the Absolute state of existence.

Chit

So *buddhi, manas* and *ahankar* evolve through spiritual practice, and with this

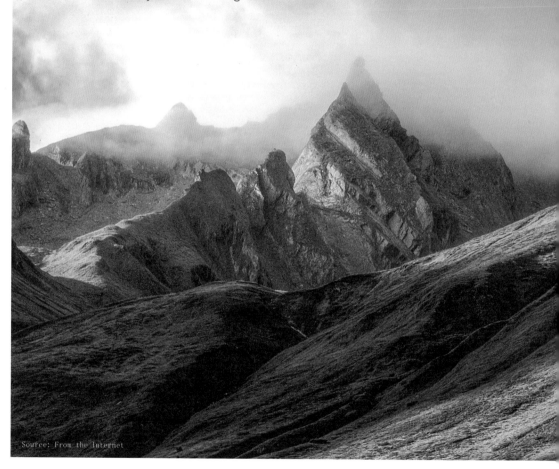

the subtle body becomes lighter, purer and simpler, like the still pond with minimal ripples. With this, consciousness is able to expand and evolve.

What do we then do with this expanded consciousness we receive? Let's say I have a particular state of mind, and I am aware that the condition is so good. After meditation, I go off to work. It is not enough just to hold that condition; I must be able to radiate that condition wilfully, consciously, and with the confidence that wherever I go it will spread its fragrance on its own.

So after meditation think for a while that, "The condition which is within me is also outside me. Everything around me is absorbed in a similar state. When I look at people, or talk to them, or listen to them, or I am silent, let that condition spread everywhere." Let consciousness expand wherever it can go.

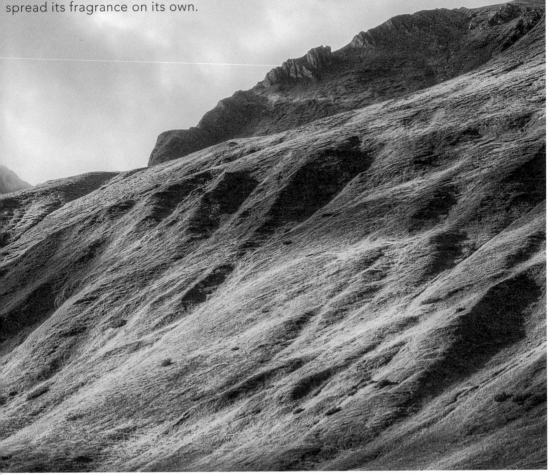

意识的进化：心灵静修旅程

The Evolution of Consciousness Series
The Spiritual Journey

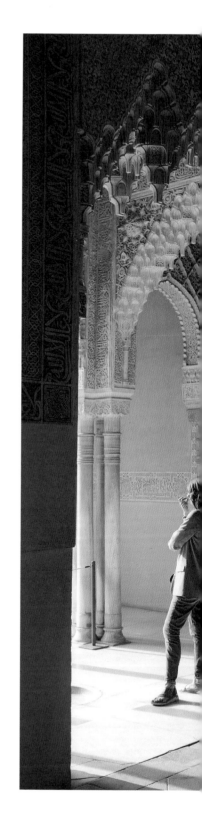

在上文中，葛木雷什·D. 巴特尔描述了人类的细体，包括它如何进化，以及冥想修习在这个过程中的重要性。在本文中他将介绍我们所踏上的扩展意识的旅程，以及瑜伽慧能在此旅程中的作用。

先总结一下，是细体在进化，并导致意识进化，允许我们改变并规划我们的命运。随着我们净化及简化细体，灵魂的喜悦会从内在散发出来，而我们就能够将自己的意识扩展到更高的状态，揭示出越来越多的人类潜能。

在本文中，我们将看到细体精炼和净化的过程，以至意识能够扩展和进化。我们的振动场越是纯洁与简单，就越能够观察、探索，并扩展至跨越潜意识、意识和超意识的范围。事实上，没有对细体的清理，就没有真正的内在旅程！随着进步，我们的自我变得越来越精炼，我们发展出智慧，揭开了感觉及超越感觉的世界，所有这些通过以心为基础的冥想而成为可能，这个冥想体系带有对细体的清理。

还有另一个过程帮助我们的旅程到达越来越高的意识状态。没有这个过程，我们无法移除障碍，就像任何进入未知宇宙的旅程那样。这个极为重要的成分就是瑜伽慧能传递，在瑜伽文献中被称为奉献 (Pranahuti)。尤其

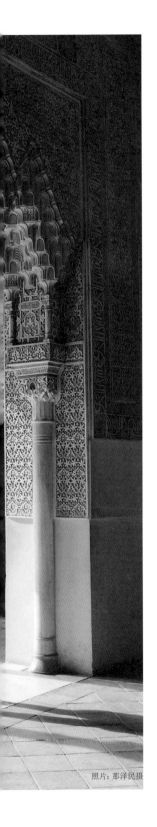

照片：那泽民摄

是，慧能传递由一位有能力的老师进行。

我们经常想象灵性的老师——瑜伽士、神秘主义者、圣人、苏菲派、僧人——他们都充满智慧和爱。他们智慧的言谈，以美妙的语言和深刻的洞见来启迪我们。但是，语言本身并非内在改变的催化剂。智慧能够鼓励和启发我们想去改变及进化，但它并不能让改变发生。

而爱能够改变，正如我们在世俗生活中所了解——爱能产生奇迹、征服一切，并让这个世界转动——内在意识进化所需要的爱是一种普世的爱，这种爱超越我们通常于世俗生活中所能理解的任何事物。在这里，师父的角色是最重要的。

瑜伽慧能的转化效果是千万年来最神秘的秘密。这种慧能传递曾经只能由具备能力的灵性老师从心到心传给嫡传弟子，现在对全人类开放。这个过程需要解释。

灵性修习的基本剖析

在本书第一篇，我们谈到了人类的三体——物体、思维和因果；身体、头脑和灵魂；物质、能量和绝对；三种主要的存在状态在物理学上也是如此——能量固化为物质，能量作为振动场，而潜在的能量处于未显现的状态。

当我们意识到这三体的中心或连接纽带是心的时候，事情就开始变得非常有意思。[1]这就是为什么现代科学家发现心的电磁场在人体处于主导地位[2]。

从这个振动的心，能量流向外辐射到世俗生活。有部分直接流向物质世界——在身体层面，我们需要能量去生存及行动，例如行走、举重、园艺、跳舞、健身诸如此类。有部分心的涌流也会直接进入存在的思维层面:思考、学习、教授、研究、解决问题,或是以任何方式进入知识和智慧的领域。

也可以这样来解释:我们持续不断从宇宙中获得的意念之流 (stream of thoughts) 来自宇宙之境,那里是万物的起源,也是瑜伽中我们所说的梵卵区 (brahmand mandal)。设想一下涌流由上面降下,通过头顶进入我们的身体。意念之流降落至心,而大多数人让其中的99%从心流到外界,被运用于世俗生活之中。

当内在旅程开启之时,心的能量流会转向内在。但并非全部,我们依然要在这个世界上生活,需要照顾好家庭,做好工作等,但已经足够感受到灵魂的吸引力。

在胸部左侧,涌流由心脏的位置向外散发到物质世界。当一股涌流转向内在时,其朝向是胸部的右侧,到达了人类的灵性解剖学中所说的阿特曼脉轮 (atman chakra) 或者说是灵魂轮点 (soul point)。这就是人的灵性之心。

这个朝向内在的运动的推进力量来自某位有能力的灵性导师所做的瑜伽慧能工作。随着持续的冥想,我们被拉向内在的宇宙,并开始将其与世俗生活相融合,这样两者就能并肩前行。

但是这种朝向内在的运动会是一个困难的变迁。这就像从一个星系去到另一个星系,头脑会抵抗随之而来的任何变化,最初会感到不舒服,这非常像我们从一所房子、一座城市或一份工作转移到另一处。这需要一些时间来适应。这本身就是意识扩展旅程中的第一个障碍。如果能够跨越这个障碍,我们就赢得了这场挑战的第一步!接

1　法特加尔的罗摩·昌德拉,《真理永恒》,2015,罗摩昌德拉静修会,印度

2　心灵数学(HearthMath)的研究成果,保罗·皮尔索及其他

下来，我们进入一个不同类型的人类意识的领域——灵魂点无比的镇静与平和……但这只是我们旅程的开始。

在下一篇文章，我们会更细致地探讨大脑如何令我们陷入世俗的问题，阻碍了意识的扩展，而我们如何通过心灵静修来解决。

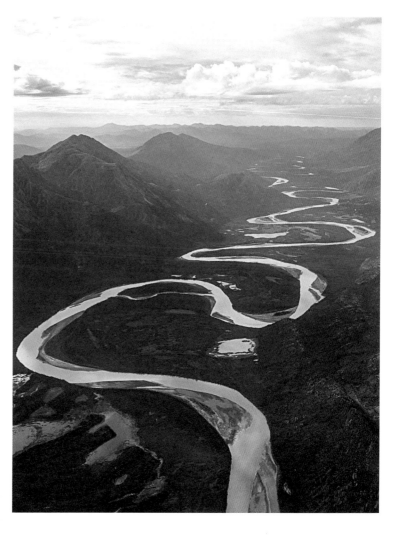

照片来源于网络

In "The Subtle Body", Kamlesh D. Patel described the subtle body of a human being, including how it evolves, and the importance of a meditative practice in that process. In this issue, he introduces us to the journey we embark upon to expand consciousness and the role of Yogic Transmission in that journey.

Just to recap, it is the subtle body that evolves, and as a result consciousness evolves, allowing us to transform and design our destiny. As we purify and simplify the subtle body, the joy of the soul radiates from within, and we are able to expand our consciousness into higher states, revealing more and more of our human potential.

In Part II, we looked at the process of refinement and purification of the subtle body, so that consciousness can expand and evolve. The purer and simpler our vibrational field, the more we can observe, explore, and expand across the spectrum of subconsciousness, consciousness and superconsciousness. In fact, without this cleaning of the subtle body, there is no real inner journey! As we progress, our ego becomes more and more refined, we develop wisdom and uncover the world of feeling and beyond, all of which are possible through a system of heart-based

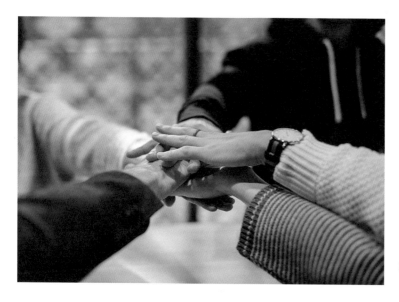

照片来源于网络

meditation with cleaning of the subtle body.

There is also a second process that aids our journey into higher and higher states of consciousness. Without it, we would not manouver the obstacles, like with any journey into unknown universes. That vital ingredient is Yogic Transmission, known in the yogic literature as pranahuti. More particularly, it is Yogic Transmission utilized by a teacher of caliber.

We often think of spiritual teachers – yogis, mystics, saints, sufis and shamans – as being full of wisdom and love. They speak wisely, and inspire us with wonderful words and insights. But words on their own are not catalysts for inner transformation. Wisdom can encourage and inspire us to want to change and evolve, but it does not make the transformation happen.

While love is transformative, as we know from worldly life – love can work miracles, conquer all, and make the world go round – the love required for inner evolution of consciousness is a universal love that is beyond anything we normally understand in worldly life. Here the teacher's role is paramount.

The transformative effect of Yogic Transmission has been one of the greatest mystical secrets throughout the ages. What was once passed down only from heart to heart by spiritual teachers of caliber to their immediate disciples, is now openly available to all humanity. And this process requires explanation.

Some basic spiritual anatomy

In the first article of this series, we spoke about the three bodies of a human being – the physical, mental and causal; body, mind and soul; matter, energy and absolute; the three major states of existence in physics also – energy solidified into matter, energy as vibrational field, and potential energy in its unmanifested state.

1 Ram Chandra of Fatehgarh, Truth Eternal, 2015, Shri Ram Chandra Mission, India.

It starts to become really interesting when we realize that the centre or connecting link of these three bodies is the heart.[1] That is why scientists these days are finding that the electromagnetic field of the heart is the dominant field in the human body.[2]

From this vibrational heart, currents radiate out into worldly life. Some are directed towards the physical world of matter – we need energy to exist and perform actions in the physical plane, e.g. walking, lifting, gardening, dancing, exercising, and so on.

Some of the heart's currents are also directed into the mental sphere of existence: thinking, studying, teaching, research, problem-solving, or engaging in any other way in the field of knowledge and wisdom.

We can also explain it like this: the stream of thoughts we constantly receive from the universe comes from the cosmic realm, where everything originates, what we call brahmand mandal in yoga. Imagine the stream is descending from above, down through the crown of the head into our system. The thought stream descends into the heart and in most people 99 percent of it goes outwards from the heart, to be used in worldly life.

When the inner journey starts, one stream of the heart's current is diverted inwards. Not all, as we still have to live in the world, look after a family, manage a job etc., but enough so that the pull of the soul is felt.

On the left side of the chest, the currents are radiating outwards into worldly life from the point where the physical heart is found. When one stream is turned inwards, it turns towards the right side of the chest, to the point in the human spiritual anatomy known as the atman chakra or soul point. This is the spiritual heart of a human being.

The catalyst for this inward movement is a teacher of caliber, who utilizes Yogic Transmission for this purpose. As we then continue to meditate, we are drawn towards the inner universe and start to integrate it with worldly life, so

2 Research by HearthMath, Paul Pearsall and others.

that both continue side by side.

But this inward movement can be a difficult transition. It is like moving from one galaxy to another, and as with any change the mind rebels, feeling uncomfortable at first, much like when we move from one house, one city or one job to another. It takes a while to settle in. This is itself the first hurdle in our journey of expansion of consciousness. If we can cross that hurdle, the first step in the battle is won! Now we enter the realm of a different type of human consciousness – that of the immense peace and calm of the soul point. ... But this is just the beginning of our journey.

In the next article of the series, we will explore in more detail how our minds keep us entangled in worldly issues that stifle the expansion of consciousness, and how we can address this through spiritual practice.

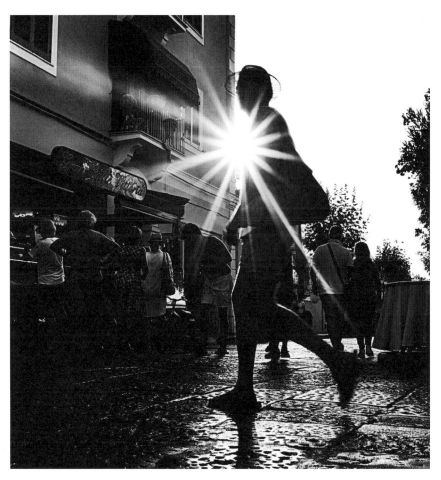

意识的进化：灵性解剖学

The Evolution of Consciousness Series
The Spiritual Anatomy

在上文中，葛木雷什·D. 巴特尔描述了我们扩张意识的旅程和瑜伽慧能传递的作用，以及与内在旅程相关的一些基本的灵性剖析。现在将更详细地探讨我们如何深陷于世俗问题之中，如何在人的灵性解剖学中呈现，以及我们能做些什么来移除由此而形成的印记。

在《细体》文章中，我们探讨了精炼和净化细体的必要性，这样意识可以得到扩展和进化。事实上，没有细体的清理就不会有真正的进化。那么，需要从细体中清除什么呢？

假如闭上眼一会儿去想象一下细体，人的心思区域是一个充满精细能量、充满意识的宽广区域。如果有助于理解，可以想象它如同一个充满水的巨大机体。当这个区域纯净的时候，它是完全静止和镇定的，就像明净的湖水。当受到动荡干扰时，它会变得波涛汹涌，而且水会到处流动。形成漩涡，产生涌流。

同样，由于日常所产生的印记，细体也会被动荡所填充。当这些印记变得更加牢固后，就会在我们体内聚集，产生粗质和能量结节，最终会凝结。在瑜伽文献中被称作"印记"（samskara），而且由于其物质性，这就是我们通

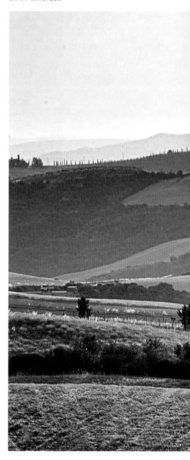

照片：王锐光摄

过降生及再降生而一次次回到存在物质层面的原因。

那么如何在细体中形成印记的呢? 让我们来了解印记形成的方式, 以及印记如何被自身的振动牵引而积累在身心的独特中心。沙杰汗布尔的罗摩·昌德拉的著作中有一个很好的例子。你在回家的路上看到一朵很美的玫瑰花正在绽放, 于是你赞叹它的美丽。下一次你再走过, 会靠得更近并更加仔细地欣赏它的美丽。第二天, 你感觉好像正手握着那朵花并嗅闻其芬芳。渐渐地, 也许有一天你会说, "让我把这株玫瑰带回家吧"。

我们被一些东西吸引, 就像玫瑰及其芬芳, 而我们也会不喜欢某些东西, 比如玫瑰的刺。我们的倾向——吸引或排斥——在我们的心里产生了一种情感。这种情感不是在头脑里, 总是在心中。这会产生一个印记。我们一次又一次地重复这种情感, 它就在我们心中形成了更加深

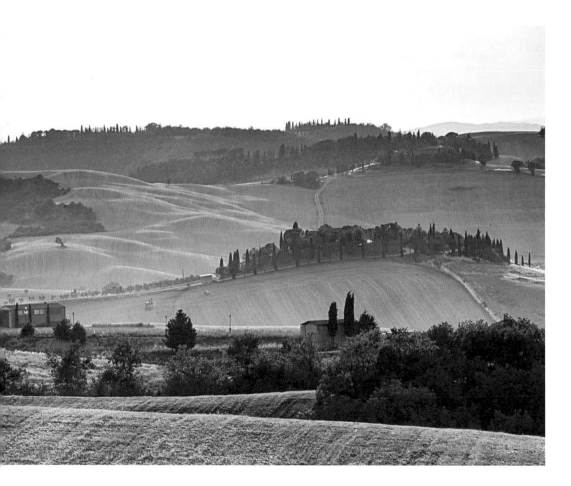

刻的习惯模式,这种模式越来越牢固就成了印记:"我不喜欢意大利细面""我害怕我的老板""我喜欢游泳""我不信任男人",等等。这些意念会影响我们的日常生活方式,改变我们的看法和决定染色。

　　在世俗生活中,我们面对着不同类型的问题、事件,有不同的喜好及厌恶。当我们持续不断地担心世俗问题的时候,就会出现一定水平的焦虑和担忧,并相应地在我们心中形成粗质。没有人能够摆脱世俗的担忧,如果一切适度就可以接受。如果我们担忧某件事,我们应该为解决此事做些什么,如果持久地为其担忧,却没有采取行动去解决它,这只会让事情变得更糟。我们持续不断地想着世俗的问题并沉浸其中,这会影响到A点,A点位于胸腔左侧靠近心脏的位置。

　　人类生存的另一部分就是我们被异性所吸引。同样,如果

照片来源于《满心》杂志

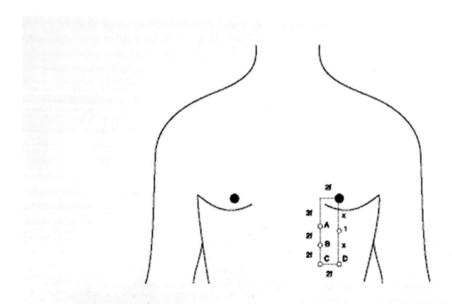

适度是可以接受的，但当其令我们感到困扰的时候，这些印记就会在B点形成。

当我们有很强的喜好和厌恶的时候，我们也将其称为对某些事物和人的偏见，我们也许不会说起它们，但我们会在心里重复，并且会影响我们的思维，通常我们并没有意识到。这些印记会堆积于C点。

内疚是我们所形成的最粗重的印记。它往往产生于我们应该做但没有做的事，或是我们不该做却做了的事。内疚会在心里产生许多粗质，这些粗质会堆积在D点。

A点的位置，在左侧乳头往右两指宽，然后再往下三指宽。由A点再往下两指宽，就是B点。由B点再往下两指宽，就是C点。C点正好在最下方的肋骨处，位于A点和B点的正下方。由C点再往左两指宽，就是D点。D点位于左乳头的正下方。

这就是这些点的解剖学位置，我们在这里积累特定的印记。人的身体中并不是只有这些点会积累印记，但这是其中最重要的一些点并且是一个开始。

分享这些知识有什么用处呢？这样一来我们能够更有觉知。我们注意到印记的聚集，就可以调整并清理自己，而不是总是在评判其他东西。

在任何个人转变的过程中，自我接纳都是非常重要的态度。没有它，我们会陷于评判之中，并且很难让印记离开；反之我们会一遍遍地想着这些印记，令它们越来越深刻。没有自我接纳，也很难培养对自己的爱。没有自爱，我们是有缺陷的，也无法培养对他人的爱。我们连第一基本点都无法到达。

清心的过程会移除心中形成的印记，制造光明和无忧无虑的感觉。这样我们就能愉快地改变自我的工作，心灵的旅程由此展开。

清心是日常满心修习中必不可少的一部分，在傍晚结束一天的工作之后进行。通过净化细体进行冥想练习。这是进行自我提升过程中最令人难以置信的工具之一，因为它移除了那些习惯和模式，而这些习惯和模式令我们陷于自己的小小世界里，并阻碍我们将意识扩展到无限的境界，而这个境界在自我发现的旅程中等待我们达到。

在下文中，我们将对人类体验的内在旅程进行更多的探讨。

照片来源于网络

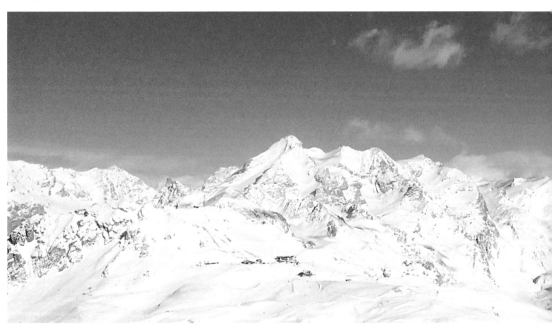

In the last article of the series, Kamlesh D. Patel described the journey we embark upon to expand consciousness and the role of Yogic Transmission, as well as some of the basic spiritual anatomy associated with the beginning of the inner journey. Here explores with us in more detail how we become entangled in worldly issues, how that expresses in the spiritual anatomy of a human being, and what we can do to remove the impressions that form.

In the second article of this series, we explored the need to refine and purify the subtle body, so that consciousness can expand and evolve. In fact, without this cleaning of the subtle body, there is no real evolution. What needs to be cleaned from the subtle body?

If you can close your eyes for a moment and imagine the subtle body, the heartmind field of a human being, as a vast field of subtle energy, of consciousness. If it helps, imagine it is like a large body of water. When the field is pure, it is absolutely still and calm, like a glassy lake. When it is disturbed by turbulence, it is choppy and rough, and

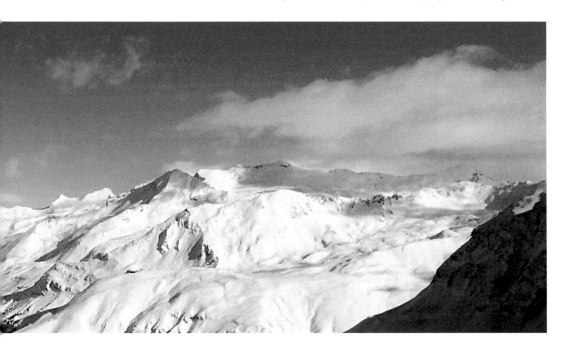

the water is moving in all directions. Eddies of water form, creating currents.

Similarly, the subtle body can also be filled with turbulence, due to the many impressions that form on a daily basis. When these impressions become more fixed, they lodge in our system creating heaviness and knots of energy that eventually solidify. They are known in the yogic literature as *samskaras*, and because of their materiality they are the cause of our coming again and again into this physical plane of existence through birth and rebirth.

So how do we form impressions in the subtle body? Let's understand the way they form, and how each impression is drawn by its vibration to a particular centre in the human system. When we read the works of Ram Chandra of Shahjahanpur, he gives a beautiful example. You are walking home and you notice a beautiful rose flower blossoming, so you admire its beauty. The next time you are passing, you go near and admire its beauty in more detail. The next day, you feel like holding that flower in your hand and smelling it. Progressively a day may come when you say, "Let me take this rose bush home."

We are attracted to some things, like the beautiful rose flower and its fragrance, and we dislike others, like the thorns of the rose bush. Our orientation – our attraction or repulsion – creates an emotion in our heart. That emotion is not in the mind; it is always in the heart. It forms an impression. When we repeat that emotion again and again, it forms a deeper habitual pattern in our heart, that becomes more and more fixed as a *samskara*: "I don't like spaghetti" "I am scared of my boss" "I love to go swimming" "I do not trust men", etc. This belief then affects the way we live our daily life, coloring our perception and decisions.

We face different types of problems, issues, likes and dislikes in worldly life. When we are constantly worrying about our worldly problems, a level of anxiety and worry builds up, and accordingly this forms heaviness in the heart. No one can escape worldly worries and everything in moderation is tolerable. When we worry about something it is a good indication that we have to act upon it, but worrying about it perpetually, without acting to solve the problem, is only going to make it worse. When we constantly think about worldly problems and brood over them it affects point A, which is found close to the heart on the left side of the chest.

Another part of human existence is our attraction towards the opposite sex. Again, when it is in moderation it is tolerable, but when it overburdens us those impressions form at point B.

When we have strong likes and dislikes, what we also call prejudices for and against certain things and people, we may not speak about them but we are constantly playing with them in our hearts, and they affect our thinking often without us knowing they are doing so. Those impressions are deposited at point C.

Guilt is one of the heaviest impressions we can form. It arises out of something we did not do but should have done, or something we did but should not have done. Guilt gives rise to so much heaviness in the heart and this heaviness is deposited at point D.

To find point A, measure two finger widths to the right side to your left nipple, and then three fingers down.

Go two finger widths further down from point A to find point B.

Go two finger widths further down from point B to find point C. It will be on the lowest rib, directly underneath points A and B.

Go two finger widths to the left to find point D, exactly below the nipple.

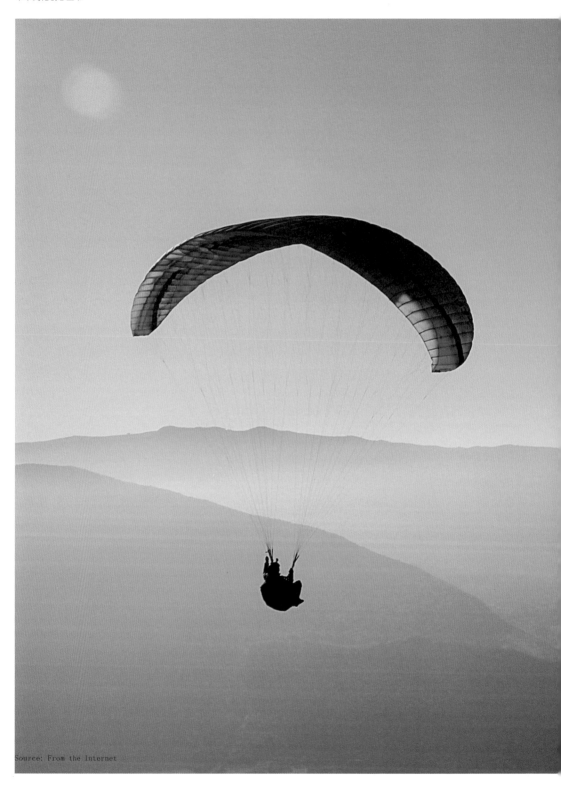

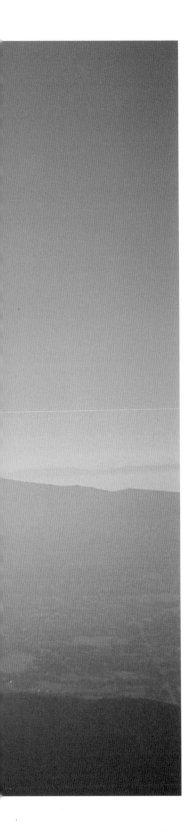

This is the anatomical aspect of these points to which we attract certain impressions. These are not the only points in the human system where impressions lodge, but they are some of the most important and a good place to start.

Why is it helpful to share this knowledge? So that we become more aware. When we notice impressions lodging, we can adjust ourselves and clean ourselves, instead of judging things all the time.

Self-acceptance is a very vital attitude in any process of personal transformation. Without it, we stay stuck in judgement and it is difficult to then let go of the impressions; instead we go round and round thinking about them, making them deeper. It also becomes difficult to develop love for ourselves without self-acceptance. Without self-love, we are handicapped, and love for others will also not develop. We will not get to first base.

The process of cleaning removes these impressions that form around the heart, creating lightness and a carefree feeling. With this we can happily work on changing ourselves, and the journey begins.

Cleaning is an integral part of the daily Heartfulness practice, and is done in the evening after the day's work. It complements meditation by purifying the subtle body. It is one of the most incredible tools we have for self-development, as it removes those habits and patterns that keep us stuck in our own little world and prevents us expanding our consciousness into the vastness that is waiting us on our journey of self-discovery.

In the next article, we will explore more of the inner journey of the human experience.

意识的进化：意识谱

The Evolution of Consciousness Series
The Spectrum of Consciousness

在《灵性解剖学》一文中，葛木雷什·D.巴特尔详细探讨了我们的情感所形成的印记，这些印记在人的身体形成结节，而我们能做些什么去移除这些印记?在本篇中，他会和我们分享关于意识谱的一些观点。

"意识"是当今身心医学领域流行的词，也处于科学、灵性以及量子场研究的前沿。意识谱并不是一个新的概念。在远古时期瑜伽士和神秘主义者已经对其有所记载，而近代以来西方的精神分析学家和心理学家，如卡尔·荣格、肯·威尔伯对此也有所记载[1]。

我们从这些文献中学到了什么呢? 它告诉我们，人存在一个巨大的意识谱，跨越潜意识、意识，直到超意识领域，而对于其中大部分我们仍不能理解。

正如在之前我们所讨论的，伟大的辨喜大师曾经说过，"意识只不过是潜意识与超意识两个大洋间的一层薄膜"。[2]他理解这个频谱无穷无尽、没有极限的本质，因为他自己的状态已经扩张跨越了那个频谱。他能够精准地观察并描述他的发现。

对沙杰汗布尔的罗摩·昌德拉来说也是如此，他研究并描述了人类心区、意区及中心区的各个轮点的意识和超意识状态。

1 肯·威尔伯，1974年，《多年的心理学》《意识谱》《超个人心理学杂志》卷七第二期。

2 辨喜大师，1947年，《辨喜大师全集》第八卷，"言论和话语"

3 沙杰汗布尔的罗摩·昌德拉，1989年，《罗摩·昌德拉全集》卷1

4 辨喜大师，1947年，《辨喜大师全集》第八卷，"言论和话语"

5 麦卡锡·罗林，2015年，《心的科学》卷2

鉴于这些研究结果，在描述意识频谱方面，科学仍比瑜伽落后许多[3]。

如果你用瑜伽慧能去冥想，你对意识谱的体验会越来越深入和广阔，并超越体验而进入直接觉知和知识的领域。渐渐地，这个辽阔的意识区域会越来越多地向你开放。

辨喜大师曾说，"意识究竟有什么重要？为什么呢？它和潜意识高深莫测的深度以及超意识的高度都没有可比性！这个我确信无疑，毕竟我目睹了罗摩·克里斯纳在短短十分钟内从一个人的潜意识中读出其全部的过去并以此推测其未来和潜能[4]"。

今天，科学家们测量脑波频率和心电磁波频率，试图描述和理解不同的意识状态，例如正常清醒的意识，睡眠的各个阶段，放松的大脑，以及冥想的大脑，只列举了一部分。他们已经认识到，心的电磁波区域比大脑更强。[5]这一点和那些有能力的

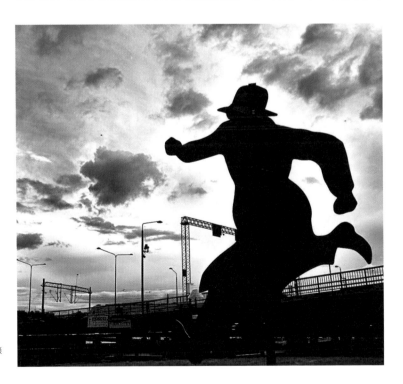

照片：王锐光摄

瑜伽士的发现相吻合,他们一直认为心是我们存在的中心[6]。

瑜伽士还告诉我们,心和脑不是两个分开的实体,相反有一个心脑区,也就是所谓的细体。[7]这个振动场从我们存在的中心——心,向外扩展,延伸至我们的灵性生活和世俗生活的方方面面。

心和脑的区域包括整个意识谱,从潜意识的深处一直到超意识的高度。在中间就是我们的意识思维,每时每刻都被整个频谱所发生的东西所影响,既来自潜意识状态,也来自超意识状态。这里总是有着一种动态的相互作用。

例如,即使对当下具有完全的意识和警觉的时候,我们从过去经历中所产生的恐惧、喜恶,仍然影响着我们感觉的方式。我们可能会对某种特定的情景感到害怕,从而阻止我们去把握某个机会,或者自己的欲望会把我们推向其他活动。所以,我们的意识思维无时无刻不被我们潜意识的过去所影响。同样,来自我们超意识的启示随时都会出现。我们或许会有一些不期而至的直觉或启发,促成我们通常不会考虑的决定。最终所有这三个层次总是每时每刻都在运转。

这种相互作用在瑜伽中被称为细体的相互作用——意、思、智以及自我。我们在第二篇文

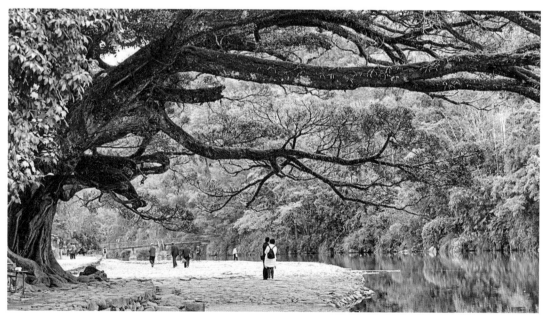

照片:王锐光摄

章中讨论了这四种细体，它们就是意识、心思、智力以及自我。它们通过瑜伽清理的过程变得精炼和纯洁，我们的意识会扩展到包含越来越多的意识谱。

当你投入地以瑜伽慧能去冥想时，你的心会打开并发展出一种能力，可以将意识谱作为一个整体去体验。这就是"瑜伽"的确切意义——整合、统一区域。你会在同一时间意识到所有维度。你的意识会扩展。

思维能够完全觉醒，处于世俗的层面，同时也深深沉浸于绝对者。这个状态就是人们所说的自然三摩地 (Samadhi)，在这种状态下，一切都能够通过超意识的知觉而知晓——大自然的直接觉知。传统的三摩地常常被描述为像石头一样，在这种状态下感觉不到任何东西，不像自然三摩地那么精细，在自然三摩地的状态下，我们发展出一种360度全方位的意识。

在自然三摩地的状态下，我们以最大的可能性去看待一切事物——前、后、过去、现在、未来——所有东西都在我们的视野内。人的意识所能扩展的程度就是进化的体现。所以，当我们在工作的时候，我们会专注工作，关注周围的环境、房间里开着的电视、办公室外面发生的事情，同时也专注于本源。我们专注于内在正在发生的转变，以及内在的状态，也专注于将要进入我们身心的事物、正在升起的念头、我们下一步将要采取的行动；然而我们在看着这一切的时候，同时依然保持着平静。

这种意识自动地变成了360度的意识。我们不再专注于任何特定的事物。当我们专注于某个特定事物的时候，就不再是冥想，而是全神贯注。

6 波颠阇利，《瑜伽经》

7 法特加尔的罗摩·昌德拉，1973年，《真理永恒》，"业"

所以在这种状态下，可以看到我们的意识能够如何扩展，并且我们可以通过这样一种动态的方式来运用我们的思维。

这里还有另一种看待意识谱的方式，从个人或个体，到整体。这是一个由脑到心的范围。头脑通过自我赋予我们个体身份，相反心是整体性的。法特加尔的罗摩·昌德拉说道："这个'我们'的'们'是什么呢？就是我们的心。"[8]我们正是通过心来彼此相连。这是我们未来的希望，而瑜伽就是开启整个意识谱的钥匙。

8 法特加尔的罗摩·昌德拉，1973年，《真理永恒》，"梵天"

In the last article of the series, "Spiritual Anatomy", Kamlesh D. Patel explored in some detail the impressions caused by our emotions, where they form knots in the spiritual anatomy of a human being, and what we can do to remove these impressions. In this article, he shares with us some more thoughts on the spectrum of consciousness.

"Consciousness" is a popular word these days in the field of mind-body medicine, and also at the cutting edge of research in science and spirituality and the quantum field. The idea of a spectrum of consciousness is not new. Yogis and mystics have written about it since time immemorial, and more recently also western psychoanalysts and psychologists like Carl Jung and Ken Wilbur .

What do we learn from this literature? It tells us there is a vast spectrum of consciousness in a human being, spanning the subconscious mind through consciousness and all the way to the superconscious realm, most of which we don't understand.

As we discussed in the second article, the great Swami Vivekananda once said, "Consciousness is a mere film between two oceans, the subconscious and the superconscious." He understood the infinite, limitless nature of this spectrum, because his own state had expanded across that spectrum. He could observe and describe exactly what he found.

This was also the case with Ram Chandra of Shahjahanpur, who researched and described the states of consciousness and superconsciousness of the various chakras in the Heart Region, the Mind Region and the Central Region of a human being. In the light of these findings, science still lags a long way behind Yoga in describing the spectrum of consciousness.

If you meditate with Yogic Transmission or Pranahuti, you will experience more and more deeply and broadly this spectrum of consciousness, and go beyond experience into the realm of direct perception and knowledge. Gradually more and more of this vast field of consciousness will open up to you.

Swami Vivekananda once said: "What does consciousness matter? Why, it is nothing compared with the unfathomable depths of the subconscious and the heights of the

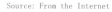
Source: From the Internet

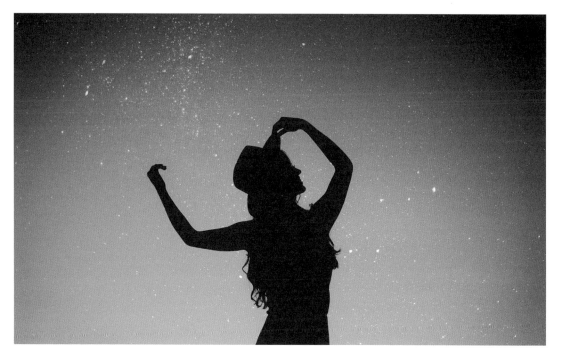

superconscious! In this I could never be misled, for had I not seen Ramakrishna Paramahamsa gather in ten minutes, from a man's subconscious mind, the whole of his past, and determine from that his future and his powers?"

These days, scientists measure brainwave frequencies and electro-magnetic frequencies of the heart in order to try to describe and understand various states of consciousness, e.g. normal waking consciousness, various stages of sleep, a relaxed mind, and a meditating mind, just to name a few. They have already realized that the electromagnetic field of the heart is much stronger than that of the brain. This is in-line with the findings of those yogis of caliber, who have considered the heart as the centre of our being .

Yogis have also told us that the heart and mind are not two separate entities, but instead there is a heart-mind field, known as the subtle body or sookshma sharir. This vibrational field spreads outwards from the centre of our existence, the heart, into every aspect of our spiritual and worldly life.

The field of the heart and mind can extend across the full spectrum of consciousness, from the depths of subconsciousness all the way to the heights of superconsciousness. In the middle sits our conscious mind, affected at every moment by what is happening along the full spectrum, from both the subconscious and superconscious states. There is always a dynamic interplay.

For example, even when we are fully aware and alert to the present moment, our fears, likes and dislikes from past experiences affect the way we feel. We may fear a specific situation that stops us from embracing an opportunity, or our desires pull us towards other activities. So at no time is the conscious mind unaffected by our subconscious past. Similarly, inspiration from our superconscious can come at any moment. We may have some unexpected insight or inspiration that drives a decision that we would not normally consider. All three levels are always operating at any moment in time.

This interplay is known in Yoga as the interplay of the subtle bodies – chit, manas, buddhi and ahankar. We have explored these four subtle bodies in the second article of the series. Chit is consciousness, manas is our contemplative mind, buddhi is intellect and ahankar is ego. As they become refined and purified, through the process of yogic cleaning, our awareness expands to encompass more and more of the spectrum of consciousness.

When you meditate intensely with Yogic Transmission, your heart opens and you develop the ability to experience the spectrum of consciousness as an integrated field. This is what "Yoga" actually means – integrating, unifying the field. You become aware of all dimensions at the same time. Your consciousness expands.

The mind is capable of being fully awake and in the world, and yet deeply absorbed in the Absolute at the same time. This is the state known as sahaj samadhi, where everything can be known through superconscious perception – the direct perception of Nature. Traditional samadhi is often defined as a stone-like consciousness where you don't feel anything, but that is not as subtle as sahaj samadhi, where we develop a three-hundred-and-sixty-degree consciousness all around.

In sahaj samadhi we see everything to the extent possible – front, back, past, present, future – everything is in our view. The extent to which one can expand in consciousness is nothing but the reflection of evolution. So while we are working, we are focused on work, on the surroundings, on the TV if it is on in the room, on something happening outside the office, and also on the Source. We are focused on the transmission that is happening inside, and the condition that is prevailing within, on something that is about to come into our system, on the thoughts that are arising, and on the next step we should be taking; and yet we remain peaceful seeing all these things at the same moment.

Automatically, this consciousness becomes three-hundred-and-sixty-degree consciousness. We are not focusing on any particular thing. The moment we focus on a particular thing, it is no longer meditation, but concentration instead.

So in this state you see how our consciousness can expand and we are able to utilize our minds in such a dynamic way.

There is also another way of looking at the spectrum of consciousness, and that is from personal, or individual, to collective. This is the spectrum of mind to heart. Our mind gives us our individual identity through the ego, ahankar, whereas the heart is collective. In the words of Ram Chandra Fatehgarh, "What is this 'we' of ours? It is our heart." It is through the heart that we are all connected. This is the hope of our future and Yoga is the key to unlocking this whole spectrum of consciousness.

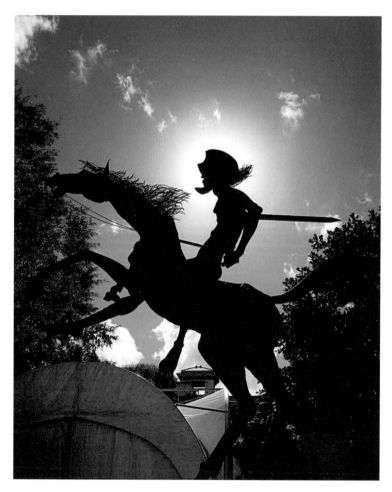

Copyright: Wang Ruiguang

意识的进化：瑜伽
The Evolution of Consciousness Series
Yoga

在上文中，葛木雷什·D.巴特尔详细地探讨了意识谱，并介绍了在这个过程中瑜伽的作用。在本篇中，他解释了更多有关瑜伽的内涵。

瑜伽就是个人的体验。在这个系列文章的第一部分，我们看过了人类的三体——身体、细体以及因果体。瑜伽作为一种可实践的方法，帮助我们精炼所有这三体，以实现人类进化的目的。瑜伽练习带来对于更好状态的体验，关乎全人类的福祉。

当今许多人将"瑜伽"一词与一套身体及精神安康的技巧联系在一起：体式、调息、放松及冥想。但是对瑜伽的这种理解并不全面。在传统的瑜伽文献中，瑜伽由35种不同的原理和方法组成，它们形成了一个完整的整体。这35种原理和方法是什么呢？而在21世纪的今天，我们如何能从瑜伽所提供的方法中真正获益呢？

四大元素

瑜伽作为一门学科已经发展了数千年，滋养并精炼了我们的身体、细体和因果体。其目的是：意识向终极潜能的扩展，以便我们能够与所有存在的终极状态合一。所有35个元素都为这个目的服务；它们并不是设计成相互独立的练习，尽管每个元素本身就包含了广阔的知识领域。体位法并不意味着要单独练习，禅

定 (dhyana) 或冥想也不是。

这35种元素被归纳为四种主要元素，也就是通常所说的四修 (sadhana chatusthaya)。

明智 (Viveka) —— 做出选择的洞察力及智慧

四修中的第一个叫作明智 (Viveka)，意思是清醒觉察对于自己进化有好的及不好的东西；什么样的起因对应什么样的影响；什么是有害的以及什么是有益的；什么是需要的以及什么是不需要的。要培养这种能力，你需要学会聆听自己的心，意识的源头。该怎么做呢?

在前几篇文章，我们谈及净化细体的需要，以便真正聆听真实的心。此外，我们探讨了冥想和祈愿在陶冶思维方面的作用，以便能够观察内在并与存在的本源连接。

离欲 (Vairagya) —— 不执着和遁世

四修的第二个，离欲 (Vairagya)，这是一种放下世俗羁绊的状态。例如，当我们沉浸于内心的满足并对世俗事务感到厌倦的时候，我们会有一种对世俗事物的背弃。我们的注意力转向了高尚的想法，会渴望一些更高层次的东西。同时，当我们为俗世的背叛和不忠而深感痛苦的时候，会对世俗事物感到失望和厌倦。当我们为亲爱的人离世而悲伤的时候，也会生起不满和不执着。

但是在这种情境下产生的离欲更多是转瞬即逝的，而非持久的。随着境况改变，它们很容易消失，因为欲望的种子仍然深埋在心中，只要环境适宜，它就会破土而出。真正的遁世是在细体彻底清理后才会出现。

明智和离欲本身并不是修习；它们是进行其他瑜伽练习后自

动出现的结果，例如冥想、清心和祈愿。当感官彻底净化后，就会发展出明智。只有当头脑得到调节及规律并且自我纯净的时候，这才会发生。离欲是明智的结果。它们实际上是瑜伽成就的基础阶段，而并不意味着成就。

除非能够自然而然地产生明智和离欲，否则瑜伽修习毫无用处。在真正的明智状态下，你会开始认识到自身的缺陷和不足，并感到心中有一种想要变得更好的强烈渴望。

六宝（Shat-Sampatti）——六种心灵静修修为

瑜伽的实用工具可以在四修的第三种里找到，叫做六宝（Shat-Sampatti），六种灵性修习的修为。其中第一种，定（shama），是指经过陶冶的头脑的平和状态所带来的宁静安详。当通过瑜伽练习实现了这种内在镇定的时候，明智和离欲就会自动随之而来。

在瑜伽慧能的帮助下，对头脑正确的塑造和调节能够轻易实现。

照片来源于网络

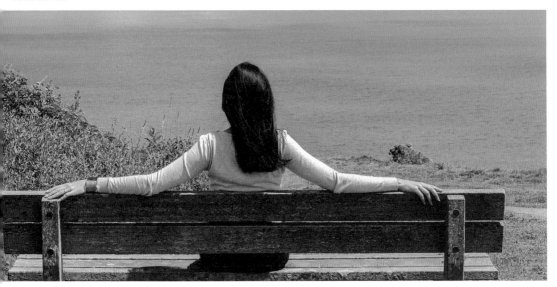

第二种，调 (dama)，即对感官的控制，通过在冥想中学会将思维集中于一点而忽略其他所有事物而产生的结果。大多数瑜伽的寻求者都遵从这个过程，而少数人试图通过业道 (karma，即行为造作)或信道(bhakti，即虔诚信仰)来达到。还有一些人通过知道(jnana，知识之道)来实现。

在满心方法 (Heartfulness) 中，对头脑的调节和对感官的控制是通过冥想练习同时出现的，自动地产生真正意义上的明智和离欲。

第三种修为是灭 (uparati)。在这种状态下你摆脱了所有欲望，不会对任何俗世的东西而着迷，也不会对下一世有兴趣，因为你的思维已经集中在"真理"上。这个状态比离欲更加精炼，某种意义上离欲产生一种对世上事物的厌恶感，而灭是吸引和厌恶的感觉都不再有。在这个状态，你的细体已经彻底净化。

第四种修为是勤 (titksha)，一种坚韧的状态。在这种状态下，你完全满足于所遇到的一切，没有伤害、侮辱、偏见或赞赏的感觉。

第五种修为是信 (shraddha)，真正的信仰。这是一种非常高的成就和难以言表的美德。这是引领你走向成功的大无畏的勇气。让你的旅途变得平坦并解决人生的问题。

六宝的最后一种，等 (samadhana)，一种自我安在的状态，甚至意识不到这种状态，处于完全的臣服。

度欲 (Mumukshutva) ——渴望解脱

四种修习的第四种，度欲 (Mumukshutva)。在过去它被高度重视，但现在我们知道，事实上它只是真正旅程的开始，因为在瑜伽中解脱以外还有很多东西。现在余下的事情是建立与终极真理的连接，并与那种状态合一。

修习的重要性

如果你探索定 (shama)，你会发现所有的瑜伽修习都能在这里找到——无论是波颠阇利的传统阿斯汤加瑜伽，更加专门的流派哈他瑜伽、皇道瑜伽等等，或是满心这种现代瑜伽方法。

波颠阇利的体系关注人的身体、细体和因果体，例如，体式 (asana) 和调息 (pranayama) 是为了人们的身体健康，制戒 (yama) 和内制 (niyama) 是人性品德和净化品格，而其他四种用于精炼细体以致发现终极状态。

几千年前，波颠阇利向世界呈现了他的实修方法，即"八支瑜伽"：

制戒 (yama)——良好的行为

内制 (niyama)——规律；观察

体式 (asana)——身体姿势

调息 (pranayama)——呼吸规律

制感 (pratyahara)——向内收敛

执持 (dharana)——精神专注

禅定 (dhyana)——冥想

三摩地 (samadhi)——原初的状态（平衡）

但正如多年来专业化已经逐渐进入现代医学一样，在瑜伽领域也发生着同样的事情，或许是因为过去每一种个人的练习和原理都需要极为专注于自我控制。也许这就是为什么今天这么多人为了保持身体健康而专注于体式。这是我们这个时代的特征，对于瑜伽的关注主要是在于身体的发展，而瑜伽对于全部三体能够提供更多。

瑜伽为我们提供了个人进化和全人类进化的巨大潜力。满心提供了一种将35种瑜伽元素整合起来的方法，而无须单独进行每一步。体式、调息、制感、执持、禅定和三摩地通过放松、冥想、清理细体的练习，以及通过祈愿与源头连接而实施。制戒和内制也是这些练习的副产品，但也会通过示意（sankalpa）的帮助精炼性格、有意识的生活、培养高尚的内在品质而实行。满心是一套完整的方法，向任何渴望进化的人提供简单的练习。

在这个系列的第五部分，我提到在瑜伽慧能的帮助下，意识能够扩展到体验自然三摩地的360度视野。而这就是瑜伽的顶点。这就是灵魂如何被滋养及丰富。当瑜伽慧能传递在冥想中引导我们的意识的时候，最崇高的三摩地状态就有可能实现。

所以，当你能够去体验一个全餐的时候，为什么只满足于一小碟前菜呢？在人类历史上，从未有过比现在更好的时刻去体验瑜伽的纯粹本质，在瑜伽慧能和瑜伽清心的支持下获得。而结果是什么呢？与所有存在的本源合一。有什么更好的方法去为我们的子孙后代创造一个更有希望的未来呢——合一和整体化。

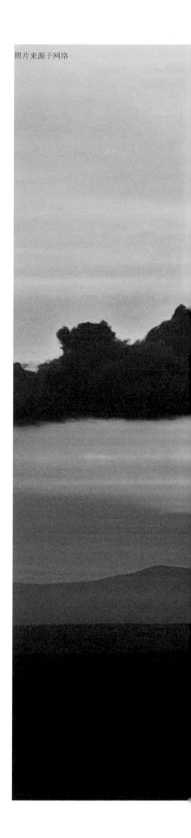
照片来源于网络

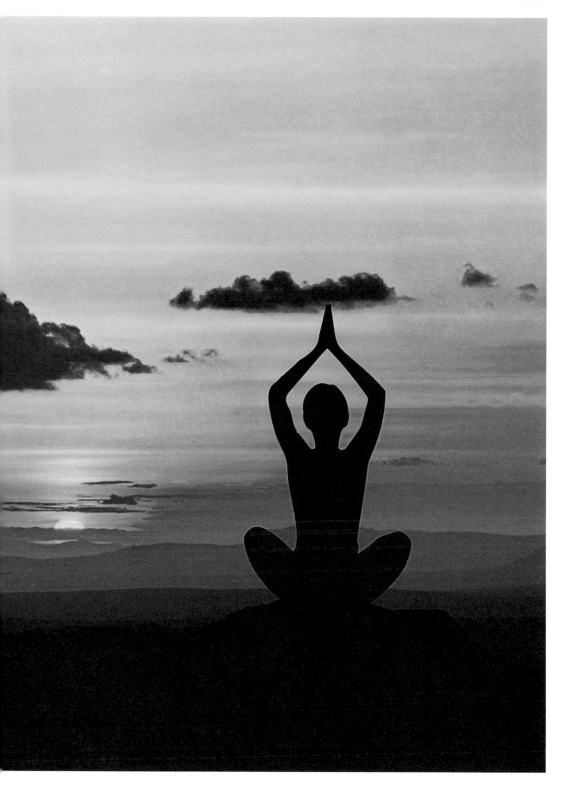

In the last article, Kamlesh D. Patel explored the spectrum of consciousness in more detail and introduced the role of Yoga in this process. In this issue, he explains more about the vastness that is Yoga.

Yoga is all about personal experience. In the first article of this series, we looked at the three bodies of a human being – the physical body or *sthool sharir*, the subtle body or *sookshma sharir*, and the causal body or *karan sharir*. Yoga developed as a practical method to help us refine all these three bodies, to achieve our purpose of human evolution. The experience of the finer states generated in yogic practice is for the benefit of all humanity.

Many people these days associate the word "Yoga" with a set of techniques for physical and mental well-being: s, breathing exercises, relaxation and meditation. But this is not a comprehensive understanding of Yoga. In the traditional yogic literature there are thirty-five different principles and methods that make up Yoga, and they form an integrated whole. What are these thirty-five? And how can we really benefits from the techniques Yoga has to offer in the 21st century?

The Four Elements

Yoga as a discipline has developed over thousands of years to nourish and refine our physical, subtle and causal bodies. The purpose: the expansion of consciousness to

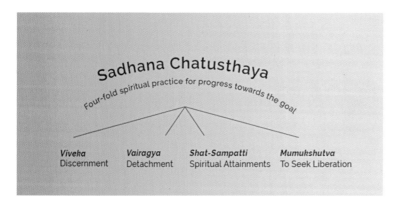

Source: From Heartfulness

its ultimate potential so that we become one with the ultimate state of all existence. All thirty-five elements contribute to that purpose; they are not designed to be independent practices, even though each one contains a vast field of knowledge within itself. *Asanas* are not meant to be practiced in isolation, and neither is dhyana, meditation.

The thirty-five fall within four main elements known as *sadhana chatusthaya*.

Viveka – discernment and wisdom in making choices

The first of the four practices is called *viveka*, meaning the awareness of what is good and what is not good for your evolution; what is the cause versus what is the effect; what is harmful versus what is beneficial; and what is necessary versus what is not. To cultivate this capacity, you need to learn to listen to your heart, the source of your conscience. How to do this?

In earlier articles of this series, we touched upon the need to purify the subtle body in order to really listen to a true heart. In addition, we explored the role meditation and prayer play in regulating the mind so that it is able to observe within and connect with the Source of our being.

Vairagya – detachment and renunciation

The second of the four practices, *vairagya*, is the state in which we let go of worldly attachments. For example, when we are fed up with worldly things after indulging in them to our heart's content, we develop an aversion to them. Our attention turns towards noble ideals and we crave something higher. Also, when we have been deeply pained by the treachery and faithlessness of the world, we feel disillusioned and averse to worldly things. Dissatisfaction and detachment also develop when we grieve the loss of a dear one.

But *vairagya* created under such circumstances is more of a glimpse than it is lasting. It can easily disappear with a change in circumstances, because the seed of desire still lies buried deep within the heart and may sprout again as soon as it finds a congenial atmosphere. True renunciation develops after thorough cleaning of the subtle body.

Viveka and *vairagya* are not practices in themselves; they result automatically by doing other yogic practices, e.g. meditation, cleaning and prayer. *Viveka* develops when the senses are thoroughly purified. This happens when the mind is regulated and disciplined, and when the ego is pure. *Vairagya* is the result of *viveka*. They are really the elementary stages of attainment in Yoga rather than the means of attainment.

Yogic practice is not useful unless it naturally leads to *viveka* and *vairagya*. In real viveka you begin to realize your own defects and shortcomings and feel a deep urge within your heart to change for the better.

Shat-Sampatti – the six forms of attainment

The practical tools of Yoga are to be found within the third of the four *sadhanas*, known as the *shat-sampatti*, the six spiritual attainments. The first of these, shama, is the peaceful condition of a regulated mind that leads to calmness and tranquility. When this inner calm is achieved through practice, *viveka* and *vairagya* follow automatically.

This proper moulding and regulation of the mind is easily accomplished with the aid of Yogic Transmission or *pranahuti*.

The second *sampatti* is *dama*, control of the senses, which results from learning to focus the mind on one thing alone in meditation, ignoring all others. Most yoga aspirants follow this course, while a few attempt sham through karma, action, or bhakti, devotion. Still others proceed through the medium of *jnana*, knowledge.

In Heartfulness, regulation of the mind and control of the senses are taken up together through meditation practice, automatically creating discernment and renunciation in the true sense.

The third *sampatti* is *uparati*. In this state you are free of all desires, not charmed by anything in this world, nor the next, as your mind is centered on Reality. It is a more refined state than *vairagya* in the sense that *vairagya* produces a feeling of aversion for worldly objects while in *uparati* the feelings of attraction and repulsion are both absent. At this stage your subtle body is completely purified.

The fourth *sampatti* is *titksha*, the state of fortitude. At this stage you are perfectly satisfied with whatever comes your way, with no feeling of injury, insult, prejudice or appreciation.

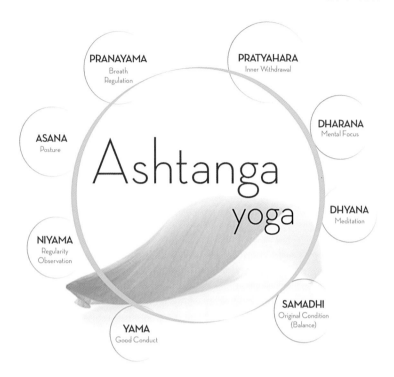

The fifth *sampatti* is *shraddha*, true faith. This is a very high attainment and an unspeakable virtue. It is the dauntless courage which leads you to success. It makes your journey smooth and solves the problem of life.

The last of the *shat-sampatti* is *samadhana*, a state of self-settledness without even being conscious of it, in total surrender.

Mumukshutva – the craving for liberation

The fourth of the four practices is *mumukshutva*. It was so highly regarded in the past, but now we know that it is in fact just the beginning of the real journey, as there is so much more in Yoga beyond liberation. What remains now is to develop a close association with the ultimate Reality and become one with that state.

The importance of practice

If you explore *shama*, you will discover that this is where

all the practices of Yoga are to be found – whether through

the Ashtanga Yoga tradition of Patanjali, the more specialized streams of Hatha Yoga, Raja Yoga, etc., or the modern approach to Yoga through Heartfulness.

Patanjali's system took care of the physical, subtle and causal bodies of the human being, for example through *asana* and *pranayama* for physical well-being, yama and *niyama* for human qualities and refinement of character, and the other four to refine the subtle body to discover the Ultimate state.

Patanjali presented his practical approach to the world a few thousand years ago, as the eightfold path:

But just as specialization has crept into modern medicine over the years, the same thing has developed in the field of Yoga, probably because each individual practice or principle required so much focus for self-mastery in the past. Perhaps that is why today so many people focus on the *asanas* for physical well-being. It is symptomatic

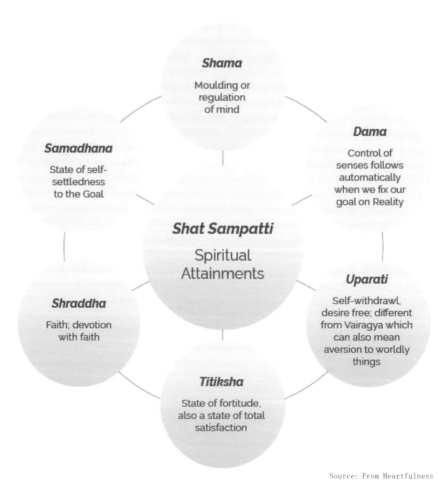

Source: From Heartfulness

of our times that the main focus of Yoga is now on physical development, when it has so much to offer all the three bodies.

Yoga provides us with a vast potential for personal evolution and collective human evolution. Heartfulness provides a way of integrating all thirty-five elements of Yoga, without having to take up each step individually. *Asana, pranayama, pratyahara, dharana, dhyana* and *samadhi* are taken up through the practices of relaxation, meditation, cleaning of the subtle body, and connecting with the Source through prayer. Yama and niyama are also a by-product of these practices but are taken up as well through character refinement, conscious living and the development of noble inner qualities with the help of sankalpa. It is a complete package that provides simple practices for anyone who aspires to evolve.

In the fifth article of this series, I mentioned that with the aid of Yogic Transmission consciousness can expand to experience the full three-hundred-and-sixty-degree vision of *sahaj samadhi*. And this is the culmination of Yoga. It is how the soul is nourished and enriched. The most exalted samadhi is possible when Yogic Transmission guides our consciousness during meditation.

So why be satisfied with a small plate of hors d'oeuvres when you can experience the full meal? There has never been a better time in human history to experience the pure essence of Yoga, supported by Yogic Transmission and Yogic Cleaning. And what is the outcome? Oneness with the Source of all existence. What better way to create a hopeful future for our children and our children's children – in oneness and unity.

意识的进化：意识的拓展

The Evolution of Consciousness Series: Expansion of Consciousness

在上文中，葛木雷什·D. 巴特尔探讨了瑜伽的博大精深，及其对于扩展我们的意识的作用。在本篇中，他提问："为什么我们要扩展自己的意识，走向更高的命运？"

我们已经就意识的进化谈论了很多，但这一切的目的是什么？为什么我们对头脑的进化这个领域如此感兴趣？为什么我们要净化自己的意识和心？

首先这是初步的基础。一个不断发展的健康产业围绕着寻找平和、内在宁静以及更好的睡眠而展开。这本身是一个很好的现象，说明我们对自己头脑的状态并不满意。我们不快乐！

在过去的五十年里，已经有许多科学和医学的研究，有关放松和冥想对人类生理和心理的影响，引证冥想能减轻高血压、抑郁和焦虑，并对心率、耗氧量、免疫、睡眠模式以及大脑的自然功能产生积极的影响[1]。

目前，有关冥想的医学研究[2]更进一步，利用最新的神经成像技术和基因组的方法进行研究，瑜伽和冥想练习对于有长期压力的人的基因和大脑活动有何影响，以及这些方法如何打开和关闭与压力和免疫相关的基因。

科学家们开始认识到几千年前瑜伽士们已经知道的东西：冥想能够带来头脑的平静和平衡，而人类的生理和心理会被明

1 https://nccih.nih.gov/health/meditation/overview.htm

2 https://www.bloomberg.com/news/articles/2013-11-22/harvard-yoga-scientists-find-proof-of-meditation-benefit

显地改变。

所以，冥想在今天已成为主流，这并不奇怪，全世界有许多公司为员工提供冥想的机会。各地的瑜伽和锻炼课程都会在结束的时候进行几分钟的放松或冥想，并且我们发现关于冥想和幸福的博客及书籍越来越多地出现在畅销榜上。

一个镇静平衡的头脑可以让我们到达第一个基本点，但这就是我们冥想的唯一原因吗？不，这只是开始。有一个平静的头脑当然很棒，但接下来你要用这个平静的头脑去做些什么呢？

人类存在的意义是什么呢？我们一直渴望得到比和平及镇定更多的东西。想象一位奥运金牌运动员，一位获得了诺贝尔奖的科学家，一位大师级的小提琴演奏家，一位世界知名的厨师，或是一个蹒跚学步的孩子。我们努力在生活的所有方面做到卓越，我们愿意为了实现目标而经历挣扎和不安。地球上的生活就是进化。每次人生都是一次进化，发展智慧、技能和态度。发明和发现也是进化。进化就是成长、改变和转化，任何怀有人生目标的人都知道，这种努力达到卓越以及打破界限进入未知领域的天性，是人类的一部分。它存在于我们的基因中。

照片来源于网络

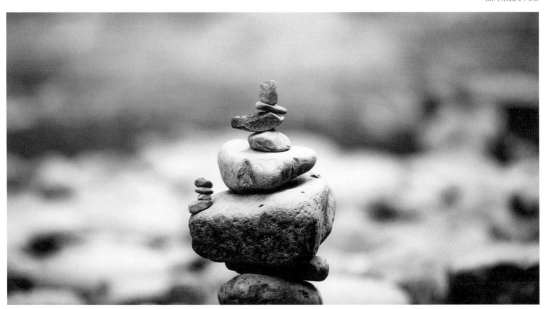

所有年龄段及文化背景的人，都曾提出过一些非常根本的问题：

我们是谁？

我们从哪里来？

人生的目的是什么？

此生之后我们去向何处？

这些问题构成了这个世界的科学、宗教、哲学、心理学、神秘主义传统的基础研究。它们引发我们的宇宙起源理论，以及我们对地球上的物质和生命基础的探索。没有这些问题，我们将永远不会发现原子结构，或者银河系及银河系之外的行星和恒星。

我们之所以会提出那些根本性的问题，正是因为我们是人。"智人"（Homo sapiens）的意思是"有智慧的人"，而"人"（man）这个词来自梵文"manas"，意思是心思，是四种细体之一，对此我们在这个系列之前的文章中已经讨论过。甚至我们对自己的分类描述也和思维相关，因此这与意识相关。

事实上，我们日复一日的生活就是为了实现那个更高的目的，尽管大多数时候我们并未意识到自己在这样做。在这个过程中，我们探求着在爱中融化自己，探求着意义，探求着逃离日常世俗存在的界限，进入一个得到扩展的意识状态，无论是通过健康或不健康的方法。

这也就是瑜伽的意义，而我们之前已经探讨过——经过各个精炼的阶段，达到自然三摩地的状态。但在过去的150年里，我们对于这种进化的理解经历了更大的转变。瑜伽冥想的修习曾被用于专注于个人向人类存在顶点的进化，然而现在关注的是我们整体的进化。这是心的领域，在这里意识的扩展跨越了存在的整个范围。

当我们坐下来冥想的时候，感觉自己的意识扩展到未知的维度，观察我们的认知进化到智力再进化到智慧，我们的思想转变为感觉，自我得到克制并变得谦卑和精炼，我们提高了技巧，这仅仅是为了我们个人的成长和转变吗？不是，这个效果会触及所有的人和事，这样我们连接在一起。不需要主动地去创造这一切，因为它的发生不需要我们意识的参与。我们就是这样去改变外部环境。它是自动发生的。玫瑰到哪里，就会散发芬芳到哪里。无论我们去到哪里，我们身上的东西就会随之而来。

我们只需要让事情发生，不去干扰这个过程。一旦我们开始净化自己，这个连接就会自动发生。然后，我们会感觉到自己内在创造的东西与整体的感觉相融合，我们将成为整体的一部分。

因此，我们的准备工作有很大的效果，在未来产生伟大的回响。我们所准备的观察者，我们所准备的区域，将会有其影响。无论未来为我们准备了什么，我们能够通过规律、良好的冥想来加速这个过程，无论我们身在何处，无论我们在一起或是独自进行。这是生存美好的时刻！

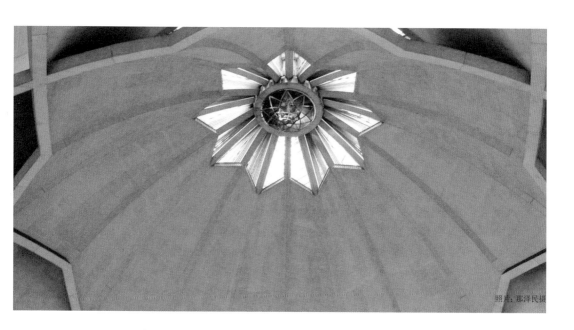

照片：那泽民摄

In the last article of this series, Kamlesh D. Patel explored the vastness that is Yoga, and its role in expanding our consciousness. In this issue he asks, "Why should we want to expand our consciousness towards a higher destiny? "

We have been talking so much about the evolution of consciousness, but what is the purpose of all this? Why should we be so interested in this field of evolution of the mind? Why do we need to purify our consciousness and heart?

Well, for a start, it is to get to first base. There is a growing wellness industry that has grown up around the search for peace, inner calm and better sleep. This in itself is a good indicator that we are not satisfied with the state of our minds. We are not happy!

During the last fifty years, there have been so many scientific and medical studies on the effects of relaxation and meditation on the physiology and psychology of human beings, citing meditation as reducing blood pressure, depression and anxiety, and positively affecting heart rate, oxygen consumption, immunity, sleep patterns, and the natural functioning of the brain. [1]

Current medical research on meditation[2] goes one step further, using the latest neuro-imaging technology and genomic methodology to study how the practices of yoga and meditation affect genes and brain activity in chronically stressed people, and how these techniques can switch genes on and off that are linked to stress and immunity.

Scientists are starting to realize what yogis have

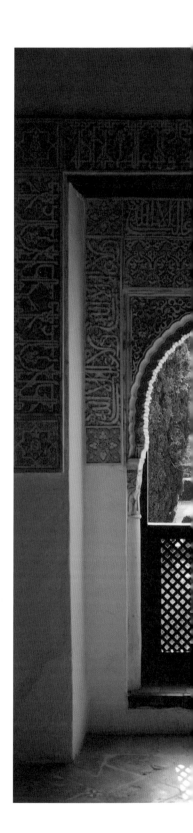

1 https://nccih.nih.gov/health/meditation/overview.htm

2 https://www.bloomberg.com/news/articles/2013-11-22/harvard-yoga-scientists-find-proof-of-meditation-benefit

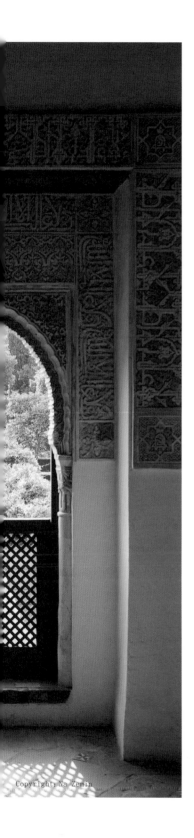

known for thousands of years: that meditation can bring about stillness and balance in the mind and the physiology and psychology of the human being are altered remarkably.

So it is not surprising that today meditation has become mainstream, and offered by corporates to their employees all around the world. Yoga and exercise classes everywhere finish with a few minutes of relaxation or meditation, and we find blogs and books on the bestseller lists about meditation and happiness.

A calm balanced mind gets us to first base, but is that the only reason we meditate? No, it is just the start. Having a mind that is still is great, but then what will you do with that still mind?

What is our human existence all about? We have always strived for more than peace and calmness. Think of a gold medal Olympian, a Nobel Prize winning scientist, a master violinist, a world-renowned chef, or a small child learning to walk. When we strive to excel at anything in life, we are willing to undergo struggles and discomfort to attain our goals. Life on Earth is about evolution. Every life is an evolution in developing wisdom, skills and attitudes. Inventions and discoveries are about evolution. Evolution is growth, change and transformation, and anyone who has ever had any goal or purpose in life knows that this instinct to excel and to push past the boundaries into the unknown is part of being human. It is in our DNA.

Peoples of all ages and cultures have asked some very fundamental questions:

Who are we?

Where have we come from?

What is the purpose of life?

Where are we going after this life?

These questions form the base of enquiry in science, religion, psychology, philosophy, and the mystical traditions of the world. They have lead to our theories of the creation of the universe, and our exploration of the building blocks of matter and life on earth. Without these questions, we would never have discovered the structure of the atom or the stars and planets of our galaxy and beyond.

The very fact that we ask these fundamental questions is because we are human. Homo sapiens means "wise man", and the word 'man' comes from the original Sanskrit "manas" meaning mind, one of the subtle bodies that we have been speaking about throughout this series. Even our taxonomic description of ourselves is concerned with the mind. So logic says that our purpose as human beings is all about the mind, and thus about consciousness.

Actually, our lives are led day in and day out trying to fulfill that higher purpose, even though most of the time

Copyright: Wang Ruiguang

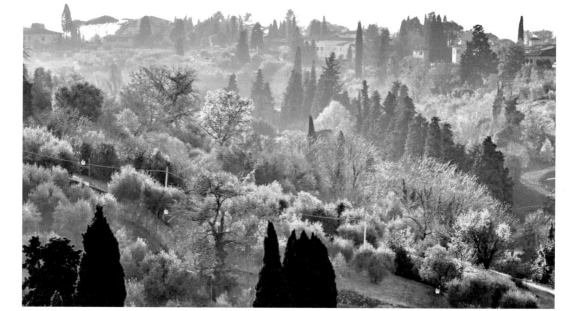

we are unaware we are doing so. In this pursuit, we search to eclipse ourselves in love, we search for meaning, and we often search to escape the boundaries of everyday mundane existence, into an expanded state of consciousness, whether by healthy or unhealthy means.

This is what Yoga is all about too, as we explored in the last article of the series – going through all the steps of refinement to the state of sahaj samadhi. But in the last 150 years, we have been undergoing an even greater transformation in our understanding of this evolution. The meditation practices of Yoga used to focus on an individual's evolution to the highest pinnacle of human existence, whereas now the focus is on our collective evolution. This is the field of the heart, where consciousness expands across its full spectrum of existence.

When we sit in meditation and feel our consciousness expanding into unknown dimensions, observe our intellect evolve into intelligence and then into wisdom, our thinking transform into feeling, our ego subdue and become so humble and refined, and our skills improve, is it only for our own growth and transformation? No, the effect touches everyone and everything with which we are connected. We do not have to actively create this, as it happens without our conscious participation. That is how we change the outside environment. It happens automatically. Wherever the rose goes, the fragrance goes. Wherever I go, whatever I carry goes with me.

We just have to let things happen without interfering in the process. This connection will automatically happen once we start purifying ourselves. We will then feel that what we create within ourselves merges with the collective feeling, and we will become part of the entire scheme of things.

So our preparation has a great effect, a great echo into the future. The egregore that we prepare, the field that we prepare, will have its impact. Whatever the future has in store for us, we can accelerate the process by meditating regularly and well, wherever we are, together or alone. It is a wonderful time to be alive!

意识的进化：时、空及万物的形成

The Evolution of Consciousness Series: Space, Time & the Creation of the Universe

在上文中，葛木雷什·D. 巴特尔从个人层面和人类整体层面探讨了"为什么我们要扩展自己的意识，走向更高的命运？"的问题。本篇中，他和我们分享了扩展的意识所带来的一些结果，包括对宇宙的领悟能力。

人生的目的就是促进可用的意识扩展，直到其充分发挥最大潜能。这种扩展最终会将我们带到一种最轻盈和喜悦的状态，在那个状态下，细体纯净、简朴、精炼，心和头脑不再分离——变成一体，心变成头脑作用的领域，反之亦然。这种综合性、一体化的存在状态，就是我们所熟知的瑜伽真正的意思。所有的瑜伽练习都是为了带来这种合一的状态，或与一切存在的本源融合。

从神秘主义或宗教的角度而言，万物的本源被称为上天或神圣。在科学领域，被称为绝对、终极的真理，或者是存在的原始状态。这是万物存在的基础，是宇宙存在的根基。瑜伽结合了人类的这两个思想领域，因为瑜伽关注的是纯知识。具有高修为的瑜伽士能够基于他们的直接体验而做到这一点，并能用科学的方法来描述上天。这种直接的觉察之所以可能，是因为通过修习瑜伽，意识能够得到扩展。

例如，在物理学中，科学家所说的时空的连续性，瑜伽士也

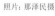

1 罗摩·昌德拉，《罗摩·昌德拉全集》，
卷1，2015，罗摩·昌德拉静修会，印度。

曾描述过相同的东西 ——梵文"空间"和"时间"的相互作用。

以下是20世纪的一位伟大瑜伽士沙杰汗布尔的罗摩·昌德拉的描述[1]：

在创造之前，唯有"空无"的存在。那么，上天的存在
是之后才出现的，而这花了一些时间。我们将空无看作是无尽
和永恒，所以我们也将上天定义为永恒。在上天之后，时间出
现了。因此空无是创造上天的来源，而时间是它的负面状态。
相对于永恒，万物都必定有其终点。而运动也存在于万物之中，
无论是清晰还是看不见。有人或许会问，那么谁创造了空无呢？
唯一可能的答案是，由于上天和万物创始的需要才导致了空无
的存在。空间是并应该永远存在，因此它是永恒的……

如果一个人在其内在发展出空无的状态，那么他就达到

照片：那泽民摄

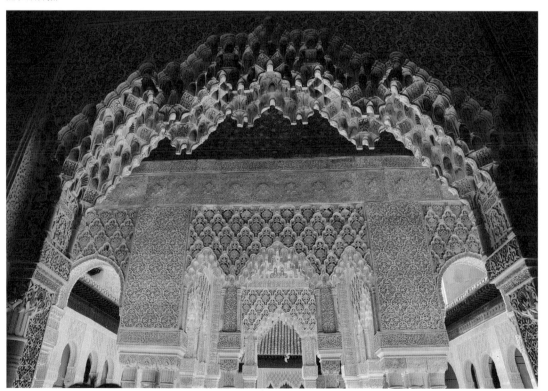

了至高点……空无就是绝对者。空无不是由微粒组成的，在其中也没有任何运动。它是完美的纯洁和纯粹的状态……

时间和空无两者有很大的不同。时间——由空无所创——可以被视为是空无的较粗状态。事实上，宇宙是时间的表现形式，而上天是空无的表现……

当只有绝对者，还没有万物的时候，根本谈不上时间。当创造的意念在基础活跃时，它还完全没有任何束缚。下面由于运动的效果其转化为力量，随着其倾向转向行动。但对于行动而言，很自然地它必须要有一个行动的领域或基础。那么，有个短暂的停顿介于原初的意念以及随后的存在，或者换句话说，它存在于因和果之间。这可以恰当地解释为"期间"或"时间"，并服务于其行动的领域。因此，时间融入力量，将其本身转化为力量，并迈向创造的进一步行动。

作为一般的原则，当一个意念加深的时候，它会带来类似停顿的效果，这种状态有着巨大的作用力。在中心的情况下，由于具有完美的统一性，根本谈不上深度。作用力速度的概念、精神的直接行动，也不会在那里出现，因为中心或者终极梵天 (Ultimate Brahman)，虽然是绝对者，但并没有头脑。

因此，存在于思想和行动之间的就是力量，被称为"时间"。相同的力量，我们也按照自己的有限能力而获得相应的份额。现在，为了利用这一力量，我们要将它融入更强大的中心的力量，那种力量是一切及绝对

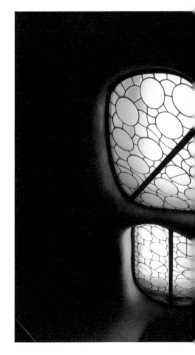

照片：那泽民摄

的……在我看来，如果无法充分认识这种强大的力量，物理学是不完整的，这种力量实际上是一切力量的根源。

以上这些描述是在20世纪40年代写下的，基于罗摩·昌德拉对时空及创世关系的直接体验而写成。他能直接感知这种知识，是因为他的意识已经高度进化。他能够轻易地洞察事物，详细地描述原子的内部结构，而不需要进行任何物理研究。同样，伟大的数学家拉马努金能够通过直观感觉去领悟纯数学函数的性质，而他的发现后来被西方的实证方法所验证。

这种直接觉知的能力，能够通过三种主要的瑜伽修习来发展，我们已经在前文谈论过。

第一是移除所有我们积累的杂质或印记，通过瑜伽慧能帮助下的瑜伽清心来实现。其结果是直觉得到净化。这就好像透过一汪清澈、平静的池水看到底部，而不是透过污浊、湍急的水流去看。净化细体的所有杂质所带来的结果就是清晰和透彻的洞察力。

第二个方法是精炼细体的各种功能——智力、心思和自我——以便意识能够得以扩展和进化。智力成长为智慧，思想深化为感觉并超越感觉，自我则放下对"我"的关注，变成为所有人的安康而存在。这些变化通过有瑜伽慧能的冥想而发生。

数学的解释：

意识的扩展和智力、心思及自我的精炼成正比。自我的负担越重，意识扩展的机会就越小。

第三个方法是通过心让意识与本源连接。这是智慧扩展的标志，并通过祈愿的练习像开关一样被激活。

　　随着时间，每日进行这三项简单的练习：晨间冥想、傍晚清心和临睡前祈愿，我们内在的能力将会觉醒，包括来自潜意识的直觉以及来自超意识的灵感。我们会认识到自己真正的潜能。

　　当今主流科学已经认识到，我们人类所利用的潜能只是非常小的一部分，但是无法给我们提供发展这种能力的工具。正是那些研究内在宇宙的科学家、伟大的圣人、瑜伽士以及世界上的神秘主义者，他们向我们展示了如何做到这一点。但是这些伟大人物却常常被形容为不科学，这不是很有趣吗！

　　事实上，在物质科学的世界也同样如此。伽利略今天被认为是观测天文学之父、现代物理学之父、科学方法之父、甚至科学之父。然而，当他活着的时候，他在生命的最后三十年里因指出地球并非宇宙的中心而被囚禁。这在今天让人难以置信，但在17世纪早期，他因为自己的天文发现而被称为异教徒！那些一直处于知识前沿的人常常会挑战现状。值得庆幸的是，现在科学开始验证意识扩展所带来的结果，而这些是瑜伽士们早已知晓的。

　　当我们仔细思考那些伟大的科学发现和瑜伽发现的时候，通常是在彻底放松的状态下出现这些研究的启发。让我们回顾阿基米德定律的伟大发现、牛顿的万有引力基本定律、居里夫人发现的放射性元素、苯环分子结构以及DNA双螺旋结构的发现。灵性发现和科学发现有着同一个源头。他们在方法上并非完全对立或不同的。

　　当我们真正深入其中的时候，心灵静修将会揭示其如此多的真正的科学基础。只有当我们不理解其意义的时候，才变得多疑，而这是非常不幸的。去看看那些宗教仪式背后的科学基础是非常有意义的，在许多文化的日常活动中都有它们的位置。

从前，这种意识扩展只是那些放弃世俗生活的瑜伽士和神秘主义者的专属领域，但今天，通过满心修习每个人都能够实现意识的扩展。这会给我们的生活带来本质的变化。

让我们把以下描述作为结束的诗篇：

我们可实现的意识扩展来自：

从执着到不执着，

从自私到无私，

从分析的反应到心的反应，

一旦自我知觉消融了，从自我限制的束缚到没有自我，

从每时每刻到永恒，

从收缩到扩展，

照片来源于网络

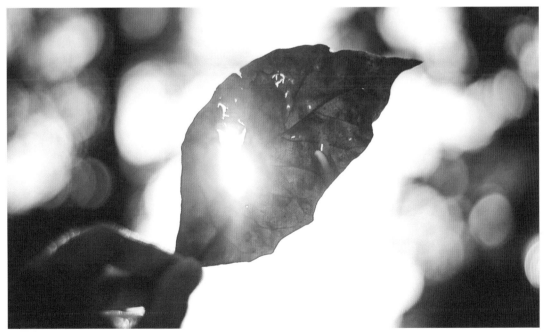

从躁动不安到平和，

从不平衡到平衡，

从黑暗到光明，

从沉重到轻盈，

从粗劣到精妙，

从复杂到简单，

从不净到纯洁，

从被欲望牵引到没有欲望，

从思考到感受，感受到体会，体会到存在，存在到不存在，

从"我""我的"到"我们""我们的"，

从智力到智慧，

从我们拥有的一切到只有爱存在的一切，

从世俗的意识到神圣的意识，

我们甚至从自由中得到解脱。

照片：那泽民摄

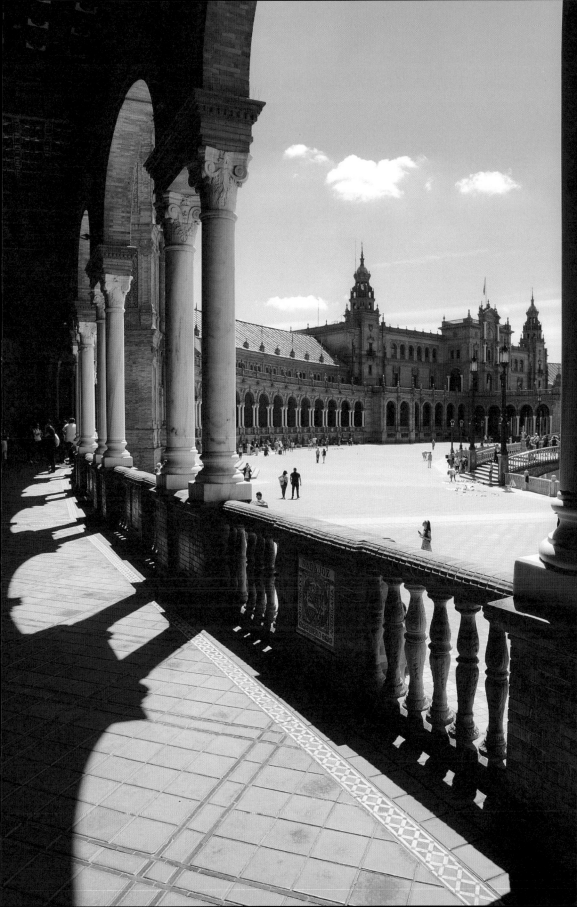

In the previous article of the series, Kamlesh D. Patel explored the question, "Why should we want to expand our consciousness towards a higher destiny?" both from the individual perspective as well as for humanity as a whole. In this article, he shares with us some of the outcomes of an expanded consciousness, including the ability to understand the universe.

The purpose of life is to facilitate expansion of available consciousness to its fullest potential. This expansion eventually takes us to a state of lightness and joy, where the subtle body is pure, simple and refined, where there is no longer any separation between the heart and the mind – they are one, with the heart as the field of action for the mind and vice versa. This integrated, holistic state of being is known as Yoga. All the practices of Yoga are designed to bring about this state of oneness, or unity with the Source of all existence.

In mystical or religious terms, this Source of all existence is given the name God or divinity. In science, it is called the absolute, ultimate reality or original state of existence. It is the Base on which everything exists, the substratum of the existence of the universe. Yoga unites the two fields of human thought, as Yoga deals with pure knowledge. Yogis of high calibre are able to do this based on their direct experience, and have described God in a scientific way. This direct perception is possible because of the expansion of consciousness that comes from yogic practice.

For example, in physics, scientists speak of the space-time continuum, and yogis describe the same thing – the interplay of *akasha* and *avakasha*, the Sanskrit words meaning space and time.

Here is a brief description by the great yogi of the

20th century , Ram Chandra of Shahjahanpur:

Before creation there was only "space" all over. Thus the being of God (Isha) was a later development, and it took some time for its appearance. We see space as endless and eternal, so we conclude God as well to be eternal. Time followed after God had come into being. Thus space served as the mother of creation of God, and time was the negative state of it. Everything must have its end in Endlessness. Motion was also there in everything, however fine or invisible it might be. One might also ask, who created space, then? The only possible answer can be that the need for creation of God and of the universe led to be the cause of the existence of space. It is and shall ever be, and is therefore eternal. …

If one develops within him the state of akasha, he has then reached the highest point … Akasha, or space, is the Absolute. It is not composed of particles, nor is there any action in it. It is perfectly pure and unalloyed. …

Akasha is space, while avakasha is time – both widely different from each other. Time – the creation of space – may be taken as the grosser state of akasha. As a matter of fact the universe is the manifestation of time or avakasha, while God is that of akasha or space. …

At the time when there was only the Absolute, and no creation, the question of time did not arise at all. When the thought of creation got enlivened in the Base, it was perfectly free from everything. It proceeded on and, due to the effect of motion, got transformed into power, with its tendency directed towards action. But for the action it must naturally stand in need of a field or base. Now the brief pause intervening the original thought and subsequent being, or in other words between cause and effect, was already there. This can appropriately be interpreted as "duration" or "time", and it served for the field of its action. Thus time, having merged into the power, got itself transformed into power, for further actions towards creation.

As a general rule a thought when it becomes deep brings into effect something like a pause, which has a tremendous force. In

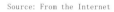
Source: From the Internet

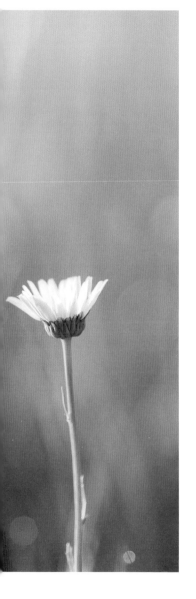

the case of the Centre, the question of depth does not arise at all, because of perfect uniformity there. The idea of velocity of force, the direct action of the mind, was also absent there, since the Centre or the Ultimate Brahman, though Absolute, did not possess mind.

Thus whatever existed between thought and action was power, which is termed as "time". The same power we too got into our share but in accordance with our limited capacity. Now, in order to utilise this power we have to merge it in the greater power of the Centre, which is all and absolute. ... To my view, the science of physics cannot be taken as complete without a full knowledge of this great power which is in fact the root of all powers.

This description was written in the 1940s, based on Ram Chandra's direct experience of the relationship between space and time and the creation of the universe. His ability to perceive such knowledge directly was because of his highly evolved consciousness. He could just as easily penetrate matter and describe in detail the internal structure of an atom without any study of physics. Likewise, the great mathematician Srinivasa Ramanujan was able to perceive pure mathematical functions in nature through direct perception, which were later proved by western empirical methods.

This capacity for direct perception can be developed by the three main yogic practices which were covered in Parts 2, 3 and 4 of this series.

The first is the removal of all of the complexities or impressions that we have accumulated by Yogic Cleaning, which is supported by Yogic Transmission. As a result, perception is purified. It is like looking through a still, clear pond to the substratum below instead of trying to see through murky turbulent water. There is clarity and discernment as a result of purifying the subtle body of all its complexities.

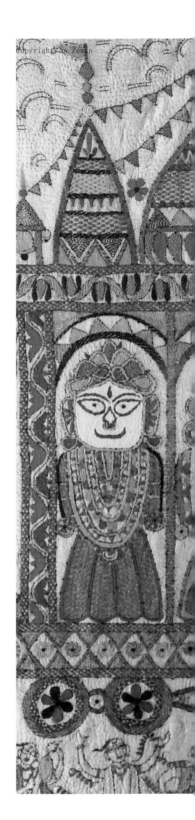

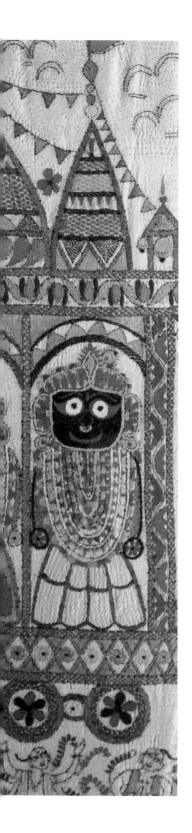

The second process is the refinement of the functions of the subtle body – intellect, thinking and ego – so that consciousness can expand and evolve. Intellect matures to wisdom, thinking deepens to feeling and beyond, and ego lets go of its focus on "I" to exist for the good of all. These changes happen through meditation with Yogic Transmission.

Mathematically:

Expansion of consciousness is directly proportional to the refinement of ego, intellect and mind. The heavier the burden of ego, the lesser the chance for consciousness to expand.

The third process is the connection of consciousness with the Source through the heart. This is a sign of expanding wisdom and is activated like a switch through the practice of prayer.

Over time, by doing these three simple daily practices of meditation in the morning, cleaning in the evening, and prayer at bedtime, our inner capacities are awakened, including intuition from the subconscious and inspiration from the superconscious. We realize our true potential.

Mainstream science today recognizes how little of our human potential we utilise, but has not been able to give us the tools for increasing that capacity. It is the scientists of the inner universe, the great saints, yogis and mystics of the world, who have shown us how to do this. Isn't it interesting that these great beings have often described as unscientific!

Actually the same has also been true in the world of the science of matter. Galileo Galilei is today considered to be the father of observational astronomy, the father of modern physics, the father of the scientific method, and even the father of science.

Yet when he was alive he was put under house arrest for the last thirty years of his life for stating that the earth was not the centre of the universe. It is hard to believe today, but in the early 17th century he was proclaimed a heretic for his astronomical discoveries! Those who have been at the forefront of knowledge have often challenged the status quo. Thankfully, science is now starting to validate what yogis of calibre have long known as a result of expanded consciousness.

When we ponder over the great scientific discoveries and yogic findings, the source of such research is always found in the overall relaxed state of the individuals. Let us recall the great discoveries of the Archimedes Principle, the fundamental principle of gravitation by Sir Isaac Newton, radioactivity by Madame Curie, the discovery of the structure of the benzene molecule and the double helix structure of DNA. Spiritual findings and scientific findings share the same source. They are not at all opposed or different in their approach.

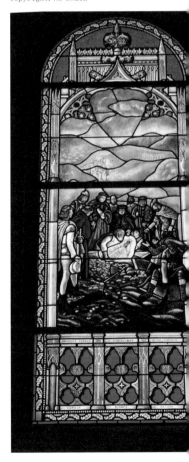

When we really go into them, so many spiritual practices will reveal their true scientific basis. It is only when we do not understand their significance that we become sceptics, which is unfortunate. It would be wonderful to peep into the scientific basis behind so many religious rituals which have found their place in the daily routines of many cultures.

In earlier times, such expanded consciousness was only the domain of those yogics and mystics who renounced everyday life, but today it is available to all through the practice of Heartfulness. And it brings qualitiative changes to our lives.

Let us keep the following expression as a poem on the last page:

Our available consciousness expands from:

attachment to non-attachment,

selfishness to selflessness,

analytical reactiveness to heartful responsiveness,

limited by a restrictive ego to egolessness, once the awareness of self dissolves,

moment to moment to timelessness,

contraction to expansion,

restlessness to peace,

imbalance to balance,

darkness to light,

heaviness to lightness,

grossness to subtleness,

complexity to simplicity,

impurity to purity,

the pull of desires to desirelessness,

thinking to feeling, feeling to experience, experience to being, being to non-being,

"I" "me" and "mine" to "we" "us" and "ours",

intellectualizing to wisdom,

everything that we have to everything that there is:

LOVE,

mundane consciousness to divine consciousness,

freeing us even from freedom.

无限的意识层
Infinite Veils of Consciousness

葛木雷什·D. 巴特尔从另一个角度阐释了意识谱，使我们对人类解剖学有了新的认识。

通常我们认为人类解剖理解是关于生理层面的身体，包括神经系统、器官、循环系统、细胞及DNA的构造和功能等。在这个领域已经有大量的科学研究，尤其是在过去的500年，我们确实对这些知识十分肯定。

但这只是人类解剖的一个方面。正如我们在之前的文章中所谈到的，我们有三个主要的机体——身体、细体和因果体。几个世纪以来，关于三体的知识一直在发展，而现代对于综合身-心-灵的科学动态领域的研究，发展得比以往任何时候都更快。因此我们能够更好地理解身体、细体和灵性解剖的动态。

例如，我们知道细体的存在是为了意识的不断提升。换言之，它们为了我们的进化而出现，并且相互支持。首先，是为了"我"的生存，为了我们的身份。没有智力的辨别能力和思维的思考能力，"我"就无法生存。思维的这些功能相互支持，为生存和发展而协同努力。

这些细体可以用于自我改善或毁灭，由于它们是思维的功能，因此可以在我们选择的任何方面上使用。具有

照片来源于网络

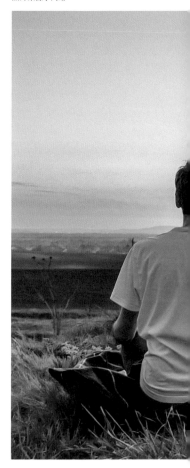

慧能传递以心为基础的冥想练习的目的，就是去学习使用它们，以便让意识得到进化。

瑜伽士也以另一种方式阐述了我们复杂的人体系统：身（koshas），包裹或覆盖物。在这种阐述中，人是由一层层的覆盖物组成，从最外层到最里层。五种元素（panchabhutas）是描述人类构成的另一种方式——地、火、水、风、空 (akasha)。还有一种分类是七区——心区（the Heart Region）、宇宙区（Cosmic Region）、超宇宙区（Para-cosmic Region）、归依（Prapanna）、归依上天（Prapanna-Prabhu）、上天（Prabhu）、中心区（the Central Region）。所以在瑜伽中，人体解剖的阐述

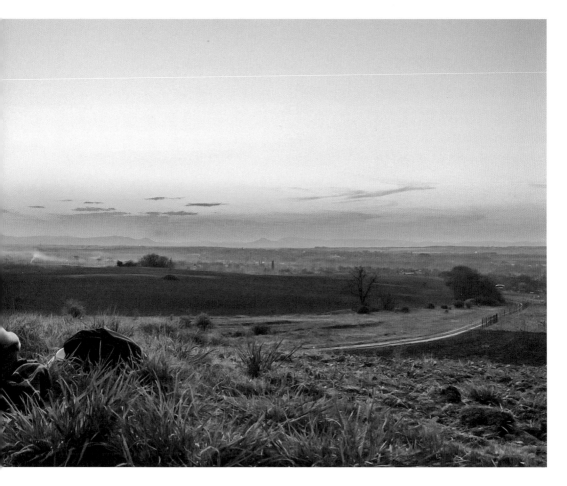

结合了所有这些东西——元素、点、区域、身体和壳。

让我们来探索"身"（koshas）与意识有什么相关。在人体系统中有着无穷无尽的覆盖物或包裹，密度最大的在最外层成为身体，越接近我们存在的中心，覆盖物随之逐渐变得更为精细。这些覆盖物折射出人类意识的无限潜在层次，这些层次本来都是我们触手可及的。它们通常表现为主要的五身（koshas）。

对于它们最早的文字描述是《鹧鸪氏奥义书》（Taittiriya Upanishad），大约成书于公元前第6世纪，在书中将它们描述为一个铺陈于另一个之中，就像洋葱或是俄罗斯套娃那样层层叠叠：

ANNAMAYA KOSHA ——物身：在最外层并且密度最大。由五种元素组成——地、火、水、风和空，我们在这里感受物质世界。

PRANAMAYA KOSHA ——气身：我们在这里感受内在以及周围世界的能量流动。

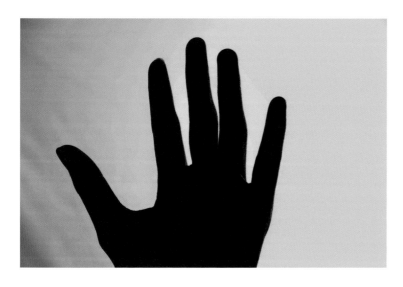

照片来源于网络

MANOMAYA KOSHA——意身：我们在这里感受思维活动——思想、意念、沉思、梦想和希望。运用头脑及感官。

VIGNANAMAYA KOSHA——识身：知识和智慧之壳。运用智力及感官。

ANANDAMAYA KOSHA——悦身：包围着灵魂的最深处的壳。我们在这里感受幸福、喜悦和极乐。

物身

物身的品质很大程度上取决于我们所吃的食物以及我们如何进食。这也取决于我们的母亲在怀孕期间如何进食、食物的质量、环境及她的习惯。这些母体的影响对我们物身的形成具有极大的影响。

当我们在一个圣人身边的时候，我们会感到精力充沛，因为圣人的"身"在辐射出能量。有一些人会从我们身上汲取能量，导致我们感到筋疲力尽。为免消耗他人，我们的摄入以及所进食的食物必须是清淡的。这就是规定适时禁食的原因，为了平衡和调节这个外身。但过度禁食会损害物身，正如太多的食物会对其造成损害一样。这与身体的苗条或肥胖无关。

食物的品质：

• 惰性食物使我们感觉怠惰和迟钝。

• 激性食物使我们活跃，但如果我们经常性或较晚进食，有时也会让我们易怒、急躁和焦虑。最好是在中午食用。

• 悦性食物促进思维轻盈、宁静及平和，并且带着感恩的状态进食具有非常特殊的效果。

执着于物身会有消极的影响，但我们确实需要对身体给予足够的重视，以便支撑一个健康的生活。物身如在更精微之身的作用下，它会发挥最好的功用。

我们通过物身受果或结束业力的影响。我们在人的物身上会发现许多变化。

接下来的三种"身"都与细体有关。

气身

气身是我们至关重要的机体，我们在这里感受我们内在以及周围世界的能量流动。它比物身更加精微和精炼。

瑜伽士根据五种能驱过程（karmendriyas）和五种能流（pranas）来描述人体内在的能量流动。

五种能驱过程是清除、繁殖、运动、手握以及说话。

人体中的五种能流，被称为气或"风"。这就是：

• 向内的流动，掌管呼吸和对一切事物的接收，从空气和食物到念头和印记；

• 向下及向外排出的流动——生理上的排便、排尿和月经，以及任何在精神层面上需要被移除的东西；

• 在向内和向外流动的交汇点上平衡和融合的流动，与吸收和消化相关；

• 向上的流动，将能量导向更高的意识层次，并通过交流来进行自我表达；

• 经脉（nadis）、循环系统、神经系统、淋巴系统、肌肉及关节运动，以及思想和情感的流动。

哈他瑜伽通常被认为用于开发气身，由于它是通过呼吸练习来控制。但能流是精微而不固着于身体的。它像一个能量泡泡一样笼罩着我们，制造出气场。细体的轮点也与气身有关，所以需要通过灵性修习去精炼气身。

通常在身体出现任何疾病之前，这种能量层就已经受到影响。这就是为什么针灸和穴位治疗作用于我们的能量经络。每当有失调或疾病发生时，首先受到影响的往往就是气身。

有时只是通过观察别人脸上的气色，我们就能够预测其健康状况。我们能够感受到不同——某人生气了，一个爱人陪伴下的情侣，一位带着孩子的温柔母亲，或是对自己工作不满意的人。正是我们的态度，在很大程度上影响着我们的气身。当气身散发光芒的时候，我们的整体健康都会受益。我们散发出自己

照片来源于网络

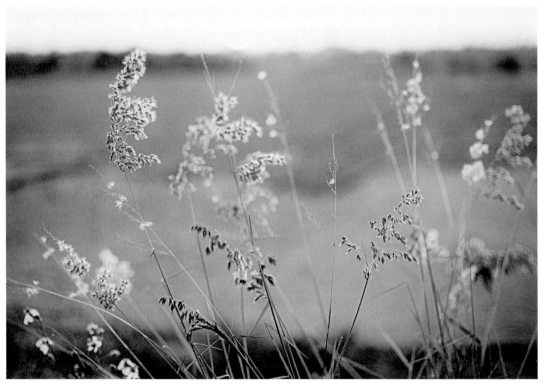

能量层的状态，包括某些状态下充满爱的喜悦的感觉；爱是非常耀眼的东西。

当我们有压力、愤怒或情绪反应的时候，需要更多的能量。所以我们通过激活交感神经系统来激活气身：我们的心率加速、呼吸变化，我们的身体进入应激反应。

这就是制气存在于瑜伽中的原因之一——平衡交感和副交感神经系统。当压力令我们的交感神经系统活跃的时候，我们可以通过左鼻孔刺激副交感神经系统来让自己冷静。当我们需要更积极主动的时候，我们可以通过右鼻孔刺激交感神经系统。我们能够实现平衡。

这个能量层是难以净化的，因为在这里意识混合着自我，而这就像金属钠暴露于湿气中一样——爆炸。我们所有的能驱过程和认知感官，都从这一层中汲取能量，我们的清醒意识受这一层调节，而本能的激情和愤怒也由这一层滋生。

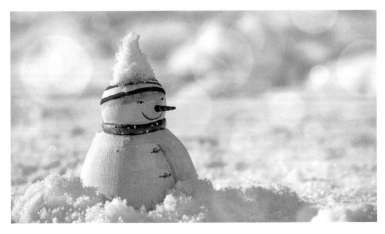

照片来源于网络

在工作场所和家里与自己亲近的人发生争执和冲突，正是由于这一层失调。当它被破坏的时候，我们会变得很自负，相反如果能正确使用，就能帮助实现大我。

对享乐的过分关注以及极度的物质主义，会扭曲能量层的精微平衡。相反，对我们的情感和所有能力的节制，会让气身和谐，这反过来又有助于物身的调和。满心修习的A点冥想和B点清心，也让这个"身"得到净化。

对立面的表现在这一层会表现得十分强烈。不断加重的喜好和厌恶、吸引和排斥等态度，都会使这一层变得更加棘手。在这种情况下很难做到节制。我们应该对言谈、肢体语言和内在态度保持警觉。这意味着要谦卑和尊重对待每一个人，包括年幼的和年长的。不断深入到一种微不足道的状态，控制自我，这是净化这一层的最保险的方法。只有当我们把自我完全净化到原本的纯洁之后，气身才会散发出其真正的光彩。

意身

接下来是更为精妙的"意身"，这一层运作于精神、心思，以及五种感官——视觉、听觉、触觉、嗅觉和味觉。这一层比前两层更为辽阔，并且全部与思维过程相关——思想、念头、原因、逻辑、思考、感觉、梦想、希望，以及好和坏、快乐和悲伤、愉悦和痛苦的感觉。

在其他动物身上，这一层基本上处于休眠状态，但是在人类身上开发得很好。这一层与心一并定义了人类的本质，并成为人类生活与神性生活之间的桥梁。

通过开发意身，我们能够得出自己的推论。我们通过质疑、体验、观察、分析、探索和推理来运用它。在我们所从事的任何事情上，我们都需要直接的经验，包括在灵性方面，为了让我们的意身能够维持功效和健康。别人进食能让我们填饱肚子吗？别人上了大学能让我们在智力上有所进步吗？

即使我们犯错误，意身也会成长。当我们努力分析问题时，有时会得出错误的结论，但这就是我们通过运用自己的意身进行学习。

在儿童教育中记住这一点是很重要的。完全建立于死记硬背的基础上的教育并没有帮助孩子们开发这一层。

甚至作为成人，如果我们只是进行阅读、观看视频、不断引用他人的观点，不论这些知识有多么深刻，我们仍然会陷入僵滞，因为那些都是借来的知识。必须去实践、去体验，才能获益。

当意身经受日常事务磨练的时候，它就会得到开发。这就是家庭生活十分有益于意识进化的原因。每天都有挑战，而当意身受到磨练的时候，意识也得以进化。所以逃离社会和问题，对我们的成长没有帮助。

挣扎和承受苦难会让意身受益，因为这些问题向我们发出挑战，要求我们去寻求解决方案，为了自己而去体验、接受并继续前行。如果我们平和地接受，这些问题会对我们有所帮助，而假如我们愉悦并心怀感激地接受，会立刻改变我们的生命，跨越到更高的意识水平。

但是"意身"也能发展出一套逻辑来维护自己的行动，不管是非对错去为我们的愤怒、不作为、慵懒、羡慕、嫉妒和错误进行辩解。当其不纯时，这个"身"会无底线地为自己满足欲望、采取不正当手段等不道德行为进行辩解。假如我们屈服于妥协的思想，我们就是对自己进化至关重要的事情进行妥协。

一名满心培训员能够通过几次打坐轻松地矫正这些倾向，将意流转向下一个轮点，灵魂之所或灵魂轮 (atma chakra)。经过一段时间的修习，我们的思维得到规整，这样我们就能够处于一种接受的状态中。满心修习中对于心附近的A点冥想和B点清心，也会有所帮助。满心修习对净化这一棘手的层叠，堪称是恩赐。

只有当我们摆脱这些精神困扰的需求时，个人的知足和真正的平和才有可能实现。当我们越来越多人加入这个崇高的追求，个人的平和将导致世界和平。

正是意身带给我们最大的满足，也会有最大的不满或不安。当其粗杂和沉重的时候，这一层会增加我们的困惑和混乱。当其聚焦于更高领域时，能够帮助我们表现出非凡的精神奇迹，包括人们经常谈论的星际旅行。

识身

接下来是"识身"，这是知识或智慧的层，运用我们的智力和辨别能力，以及五种感官认知。随着这个层的净化，我们的智力会扩展到包括智力、直觉、智慧以及之外的东西。有时它被描述为"见证的思维"，因为这时意识不再陷入我们的思想、情绪

照片来源于网络

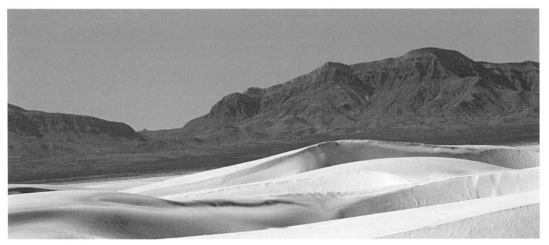

和行动中，所以它能够见证任何事物。

识身比之前的三种身都更加精微，并且在之前同类层叠的基础上，能够去认知和重新认知。当达到最佳时，它能够保持与最高意识的和谐一致。至少它能指导我们分辨什么是暂时的以及什么是永恒的。这种智慧在灵性上是必不可少的。当这种洞察的状态发展成熟的时候，我们会自动地发展到不再执着于暂时的事物，导致一种其结果是一种"不依附的连接"状态。这时思维能够保持活跃参与日常活动；关键在于怀着这样的信念，即不是我们在做。如果我们允许自己的创造者来处理我们所从事的任何行动，那么我们就摆脱了依附。

"识身"与自我知觉最为相关。通过这一层，我们的意识能够扩展到超意识的天空，以及潜意识的深处。随着这个层变得越来越精炼，它帮助我们到达更加精微的超意识层次。在这里值得再次强调的是，正是在有慧能传递的冥想修习的帮助下，这样的扩展才成为可能。

"识身"也有助于我们决定任何行动方案。基于之前类似的情况，我们学会做出明智的选择，例如，不要玩蛇，不要把手放在火上，等等。大脑接收到类似的境况，意识将记忆(认知)注入，而智力和智慧则帮助我们作出选择。

当这种辨识导致了正确和有利的结果时，我们变得更加有信心。当未能产生有利的结果时，我们会失去信心。然后，我们回头检查自己的过程，看看在哪里出错。回溯的这一步，对于持续进行自我提升非常重要。到一定的时候，我们学会倾听内心。有时心告诉我们要避免某些事情，但我们不理，然后我们看到了后果，导致遗憾。没关系!不要再重犯。

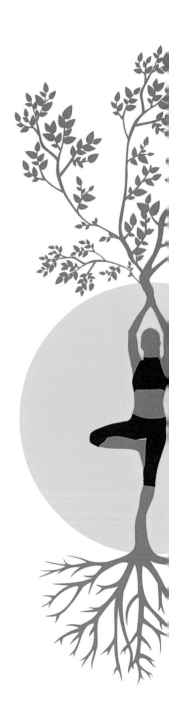

照片来源于网络

满心冥想加速净化各种"身"、诸轮点，以及整个身体的振动水平。与细体相关的这三种"身"的帮助对于任何工作来说，都是有用的资产。当持续向内关注心的时候，它们会表现得最好，于是心就成了指引。一颗天真纯洁的心会有所帮助。值得提起主基督的话："要像小孩子一样。"那种孩子般的状态反映着天真纯洁。儿童不会带着自我去说："我都知道。"这样的说法阻碍了意识的扩展。

细体及其相关三种"身"的组合协作，对于印记、思想、记忆以及类似的回忆的形成和消融，也扮演着重要的角色，因此在需要的时候提供信息。

悦身

那么，最后我们有悦身，包裹着灵魂或者因果体，与之相关的是一个更加精微的意识层次。这是幸福、喜悦和极乐的层，它的食粮就是愉悦。这一层超越了知识和体验，超越了思维。与"存在"相关，在那里我们就是极乐。

悦身是这五种"身"之中最为精微的。在我们的旅程中，我们跨越了不同的灵性状态，给我们带来了不同层次的体验，越来越多地展现我们的意识。我们在其他四种"身"的层次上所表现的喜悦，有赖于悦身所产生的共振。甚至第五种"身"也不是旅程的终点，尽管存在–意识–极乐 (sat-chit-anand) 被认为是如此高的状态。

在灵性旅程中，所有这些都要超越。这种超越是人类进化旅程的另一种描述，意识的扩展。

所有的"身"都有其固有局限性，无论它们有多么精微。事实上，它们是交织在一起的，和木制的俄罗斯套娃不同，并不是

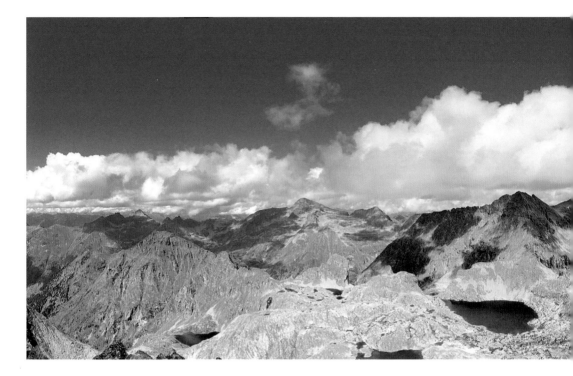

一个接一个严格按顺序排列。在冥想中，我们经常会有杂念。根据我们杂念的种类，我们可以推断出我们各种"身"所受到的多或少的局限。

所以细体和"身"之间有如下的对应关系：

Ahankar，自我，是意志力和生命力的细体，与气身的关系最密切。

Manas，思，思维，与意身的关系最密切

buddhi，智，与识身的关系最密切。

那么意（chit），意识又如何呢？还记得意识就像画布，其他三种细体在上面发挥功效，所以它与细体的三种"身"都关系密切——气身、意身、识身。但是意识也存在于外在身体的每个器官和每个细胞当中，而在这个谱系的另一端，它与灵魂也最为接近。那么它在哪儿呢？

意识无处不在。对于一个完全觉悟的瑜伽士来说，意识是360度的，在有需要的时候流

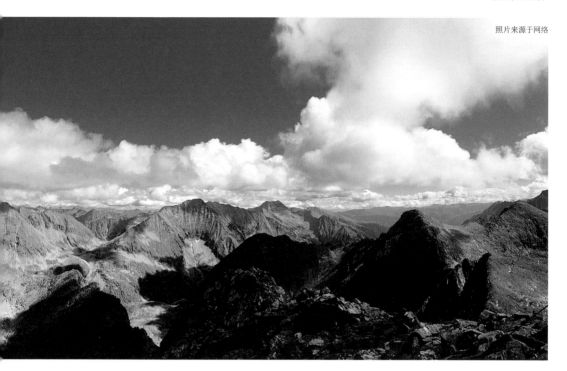

向任何地方。意识遍及人的所有"身"。

即使我们还未完全开悟，也认识不到我们意识所能到达的全部，这仅仅是因为我们没有让意识扩展到潜意识和超意识的整个谱系。"身"是以另一种方式去描述意识谱，也就是随着我们旅程越来越深入而扩展的意识谱。

瑜伽就是为了这个目的——通过系列的修习来净化我们的能量中心或轮点，净化包裹物或"身"，并帮助我们跨越意识的不同层次。

根据意识在五"身"错综复杂的网络上的表现，我们每个人都展现出不同的意识，这会通过冥想和清心的修习得到净化。慧能传递 (pranahuti) 极大加快了这个净化过程。当我们能够在将自己的意识在所有这五"身"和谐，我们将会看到生命的喜悦自然流淌。

Kamlesh D. Patel describes the spectrum of consciousness from another perspective, giving us a new level of understanding about our subtle human anatomy.

Generally we think of human anatomy as being about the physical body, including the nervous system, the organs, the circulatory system, the structure and functioning of cells and DNA, etc. There has been so much scientific research in this field, especially during the last 500 years; we have really specialized in this knowledge.

But this is only one aspect of human anatomy. As we have discussed in previous articles, we have three main bodies – the physical, subtle and causal. Over the centuries, the knowledge of these three bodies has developed, and today research in the dynamic field of integrative body-mind-spirit science is unfolding faster than ever before. So we are better able to understand the dynamics of the physical, subtle and spiritual anatomies. This is the juncture of science and spirituality.

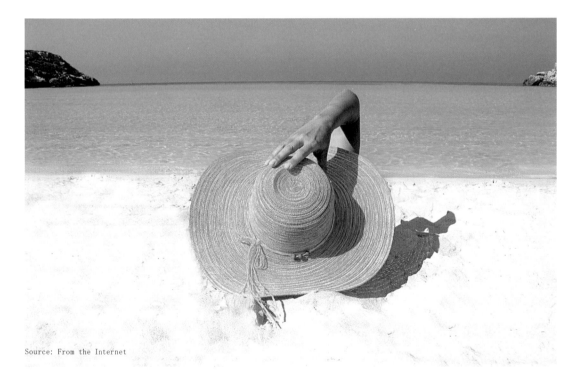

Source: From the Internet

For example, we know that the subtle bodies came into existence for the continuous improvement of consciousness. In other words, they arose for our evolution, and they support each other. First of all it was for the survival of the "I", for our identity. The "I" could not survive without the discrimination of the intellect and the thinking capacity of the mind. These functions of the mind support each other in a coordinated effort for existence and growth.

These subtle bodies can be used for our betterment or for our undoing, as they are functions of the mind that can be used in any way we choose. The purpose of a heartbased meditation practice with transmission is to learn to use them so that consciousness evolves.

Yogis also describe our complex human system in another way: the koshas, sheaths or coverings. In this description, a human being is made up of layer upon layer of coverings, from the outermost to the innermost. The five elements, or pancha bhutas, are yet another way of describing the human make-up – earth, fire, water, air and ether (akasha). Still another classification is that of the seven regions – the Heart Region, Cosmic Region, Paracosmic Region, Prapanna, Prapanna-Prabhu, Prabhu and the Central Region. So in Yoga, a description of human anatomy combines all these things – the elements, points, regions, bodies and sheaths.

Let's explore what the koshas tell us about consciousness. There are an infinite number of coverings or sheaths in the human system, the densest being the physical at the outside, with progressively finer and finer coverings as we approach the center of our being. They are indicators of the infinite layers of consciousness we potentially have at our disposal. They are usually presented as five main koshas.

The first text describing them is the Taittiriya Upanishad, written around the 6th century BCE, where they are described as lying one inside the other, like the layers of an onion or Russian matryoshka dolls:

• ANNAMAYA KOSHA – PHYSICAL SHEATH: Outermost and densest. Combination of the five elements – earth, fire, water, air and ether (akasha). Where we experience the world of matter.

• PRANAMAYA KOSHA – ENERGY SHEATH: Where we experience the flow of energy within, and with the world around us.

• MANOMAYA KOSHA – MENTAL SHEATH: Where we experience mental activities – thoughts, ideas, reflections, dreams and hopes. Makes use of the mind and the sense organs.

• VIGNANAMAYA KOSHA – WISDOM SHEATH: Knowledge and wisdom sheath. Makes use of the intellect and the sense organs.

• ANANDAMAYA KOSHA – BLISS SHEATH: Innermost sheath around the soul. Here we experience happiness, joy and bliss.

PHYSICAL SHEATH

The quality of the annamaya kosha depends a lot on the type of food we eat and how we eat it. It also depends on how our mother ate during pregnancy, the quality of that food, the environment, and her habits. These maternal influences contribute heavily towards the make up of our annamaya kosha.

When we are in the company of a saint we feel energetic, because the kosha of the saint is radiating energy. There are some other people who draw energy from us, so that we feel drained. To avoid draining others, our intake of food and the quality of the food we eat must be light. That is why fasting is prescribed now and then, to balance and regulate this kosha. But too much fasting can damage the annamaya kosha, just as too much food can damage it. This is not related to having a lean or a heavy body.

Regarding the quality of food:

• Tamasic foods make us feel lazy and lethargic,

• Rajasic foods make us active, but also sometimes irritable, short-tempered and anxious, if we eat them too often and late in the day. They are best eaten around noon,

• Sattvik foods promote lightness, calmness and peace of mind, and

• Food consumed with gratefulness has a very special impact.

A preoccupation with this sheath can have a negative effect, but we do need to pay enough attention to the body to support a healthy life. It functions best when it is under the influence of the subtler koshas.

The annamaya kosha is one kosha where we undergo or play out the effect of karma. We find a lot of variation in the physical sheaths of people.

The next three koshas are all associated with the subtle bodies:

ENERGY SHEATH

The pranamaya kosha is our vital body, where we experience the flow of energy in our system, and with the world around us. It is subtler and more refined than the annamaya kosha.

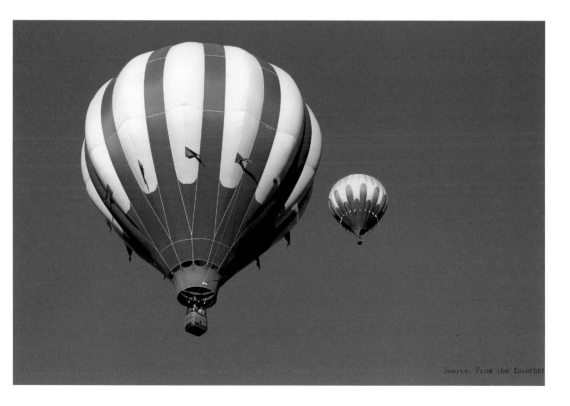

Source: From the Internet

Yogis have described the energy flow in the human system according to five energetic processes (karmendriyas) and five energy flows (pranas).

The five energetic processes are elimination, reproduction, movement, grasping with our hands, and speaking.

The five flows of energy within the human body are known as the vayus or "winds". These are:

• The inward flow that governs respiration and the reception of everything, from air and food to ideas and impressions,

• The downward and outward flow of elimination – excretion, urination and menstruation on the physical level, and anything that needs to be removed mentally,

• The balancing and integrating flow at the meeting point between the inward and outward flows, associated with assimilation and digestion,

• The ascending flow that directs energy towards higher levels of consciousness and governs self-expression through communication, and

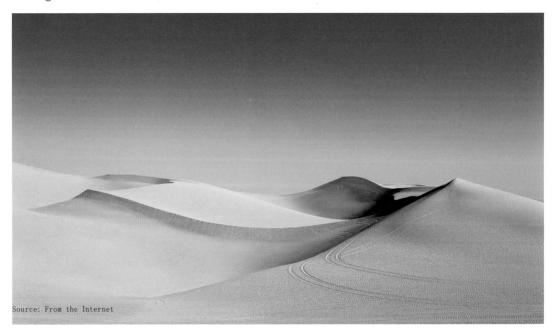

Source: From the Internet

• The flow through the nadis, the circulatory system, the nervous system, the lymphatic system, the movement of muscles and joints, and thoughts and emotions.

Hatha yoga is often prescribed to develop this kosha, as it is regulated by breathing exercises. But the sheath of prana is subtle and not glued to the physical system. It envelops us like an energy bubble, creating the field of the aura. The chakras of the subtle body are also associated with this kosha, so spiritual practices are needed to refine the pranamaya kosha.

This energy sheath is usually affected before any physical ailment appears in the body. That is why acupuncture and acupressure treatments work on our energy meridians. Whenever an imbalance or illness happens, the first kosha to be compromised is often the pranamaya kosha.

Sometimes we can predict the health of a person just by looking at the aura around their face. We feel the difference – someone is angry, a lover in the company of her beloved, a tender mother with her baby, or someone not happy about the work they are doing. It is our attitude that affects our pranamaya kosha to a large extent. When this kosha is shining, our overall health is benefited. We radiate whatever state we have in our energy sheath, including a loving joyous feeling in certain situations; love is something very palpable.

When we are stressed, angry, or emotionally reactive, we need more energy. So we activate the pranamaya kosha by activating the sympathetic nervous system: our heart rate goes up, our breathing changes, and our body goes into its stress response.

This is one of the reasons why pranayama came into being in Yoga – to balance the sympathetic and parasympathetic systems. When our sympathetic nervous system is activated by stress, we can calm ourselves by activating the parasympathetic system through the Chandra nadi. And when we need to be more active and engaged, we can activate the sympathetic system through the Surya nadi. We are able to bring about balance.

This energy kosha is quite forbidding to refine, because here consciousness mixes with ego, and that can be like sodium metal exposed to moisture – explosive. All our energetic processes and cognitive senses derive their energy from this sheath, our waking consciousness is regulated by this sheath, and the natural emotions of passion and anger are nourished by this sheath.

Fights and conflicts at work and at home with dear ones are due to the maladjustment of this sheath. When it is spoilt, we can be terribly egotistical whereas if rightly used it supports Self-Realization.

Obsessive attention to pleasure as well as excessive materialism can distort the finer balance of the energy sheath. In contrast, moderation of our emotions and all our faculties harmonizes the pranamaya kosha, and this in turn helps to harmonize the annamaya kosha. The Heartfulness practices of meditation on point A and cleaning of point B also refine this kosha.

The play of opposites is very strong with this sheath. The ever-weighing attitudes of likes and dislikes, attraction and repulsion, make this sheath even more formidable. Moderation is hard to come by when such is the case. We have to remain vigilant with speech, body language, and inner attitude. It means being humble and respectful towards everyone, including young ones and elders. Constantly delving into a state of insignificance, curbing the ego, is the surest way to refine this sheath. It finds its true luster only after we have totally refined the ego to its original purity.

MENTAL SHEATH

The next sheath is the even subtler manomaya kosha, the mental sheath that makes use of the mind, manas, and the five cognitive sense organs – sight, hearing, touch, smell and taste. It is vaster than the previous two and is all about mental processes – thoughts, ideas, reason, logic, contemplation, feelings, dreams, hopes, and the feelings of good and bad, joy and sorrow, pleasure and pain.

While the manomaya kosha is largely dormant in other animals, it is well developed in humans. This kosha defines our human species, along with the heart, and is the bridge between human life and divine life.

By developing this kosha, we are able to arrive at our own conclusions. We exercise it by questioning, experiencing, observing, analyzing, exploring and inferring. We need direct experience in anything we do, including spirituality, for our manomaya kosha to remain functional and healthy. Will our hunger be satisfied by someone else eating? Will we grow mentally by someone else attending college on our behalf?

The manomaya kosha grows even when we make mistakes. When we make efforts to analyze things, we sometimes come to wrong conclusions, but that is how we learn, by exercising our manomaya kosha.

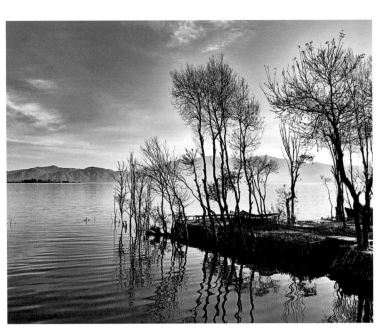

It is important to remember this in the education of children. When an education system is based solely on rote learning, we are not helping children develop this sheath.

Even as adults, we will also remain stuck if we only read, watch videos and go on quoting other people, no matter how profound the knowledge, because it is all borrowed knowledge. It must be applied practically and experienced for it to have any benefit.

The manomaya kosha develops when it is challenged by day-to-day events. That is why family life is good for the evolution of consciousness. There are challenges every day, and consciousness evolves when the manomaya kosha is challenged. So running away from society and problems does not help us grow.

Struggles and sufferings benefit this kosha, as they challenge us to find solutions, experience things for ourselves, accept and move forward. They help us if we accept them graciously, and they change our lives instantly, with a quantum leap into a higher level of consciousness, if we accept them cheerfully and with gratitude.

Source: From the Internet

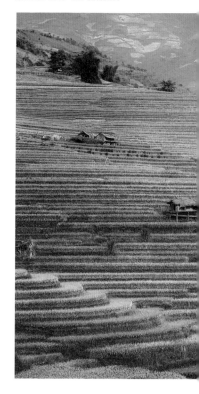

But the manomaya kosha can also develop logic to defend our actions, whether right or wrong, justifying our anger, inactions, lethargy, envy, jealousy and mistakes. When it is not pure, this kosha will condescend to any extent to justify moral turpitude for the sake of fulfilling desires, resorting to unjust means. If we succumb to a compromised mind, we compromise what is vital for our evolution.

A Heartfulness trainer can easily set such tendencies right in a few sessions by diverting the flow of thoughts towards the next chakra, the seat of the soul or atma chakra. Over a period of time, and with practice, our thoughts are regulated so that we remain in a state of acceptance. The Heartfulness practices of meditation on point A and cleaning of point B around the heart also help.1 Heartfulness practices are such a boon in refining this troublesome sheath.

Individual contentment and true peace are possible only when we are freed from the demands of these mental disturbances. And when more and more of us join in this ennobling endeavor, individual peace will lead to world peace.

It is the manomaya kosha that offers us the most satisfaction as well the greatest discontent or restlessness. When unrefined and heavy, this sheath adds to our confusion and disasters. When its focus is in the higher realms, it helps us perform extraordinary mental marvels, including the much- talked-about astral travels.

WISDOM SHEATH

Next is the vignanamaya kosha, the sheath of knowledge or the wisdom sheath, which makes use of our intelligence and discriminative abilities (buddhi), and the five cognitive senses. As this sheath is refined, our intellect expands to encompass intelligence, intuition, wisdom and beyond. It is sometimes described as the 'witness mind', because here consciousness is no longer entangled in our thoughts, emotions and actions, so it can witness everything.

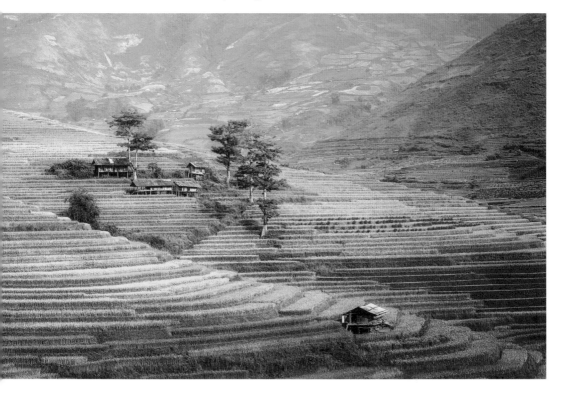

It is subtler than the previous three sheaths, and based on previous cognates is able to become cognizant and to recognize. At its best, it remains in tune with the highest consciousness. At the very least, it guides us to discriminate between what is ephemeral and what is eternal. This wisdom is needed in spirituality. When this state of discernment matures, we automatically develop non-attachment to temporary things, resulting in a state of unattached-attachment. The mind can remain actively involved in daily activities; the trick is to have the conviction that we are not the doer. If we allow our Maker to be the performer of any act we do, then we are free of attachment.

The vignanamaya kosha is mostly about self- awareness. Through this sheath our consciousness can expand into the sky of superconsciousness and the depths of subconsciousness. As this sheath becomes more and more refined, it helps us access finer levels of superconsciousness. Once again it is worth mentioning here that it is the practice of meditation with the aid of Transmission that makes such an expansion possible.

This kosha also helps us to decide on any course of action. Based on previous cognates, we learn to choose

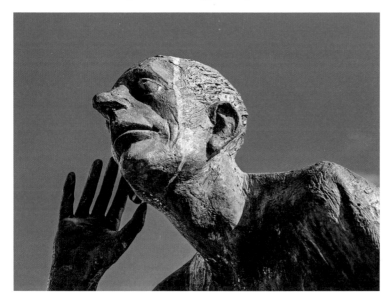

Source: From the Internet

wisely, for example, not to play with snakes, not to put our hand in the fire, etc. The mind receives the cognates, consciousness feeds us with memory (recognition), and intelligence and wisdom help us to choose.

When this discernment results in right and favorable results, we become more confident. When it fails to yield favorable results, we lose confidence. Then we retrace our steps and see where we went wrong. This step of back tracking is important for continuous self-improvement. In due course we learn to listen to the heart. At times the heart tells us to avoid something but we don't listen, and then we see the consequences, resulting in regret. Never mind! Let it not repeat.

Heartfulness meditation accelerates the purification of the koshas, the chakras, and the overall physical system at a vibratory level. The help of the three koshas associated with the subtle bodies is an asset in any pursuit. They perform at their best when there is constant inward attention towards the heart, so that the heart becomes the guide. An innocent pure heart is helped. It is worth recalling the statement of Lord Christ: "Be ye like little children." That childlike state reflects innocence and purity. Children have no ego to say, "I know it all." Such claims prevent the expansion of consciousness.

The trio of subtle bodies and their associated koshas also play a major role in the formation and dissolution of samskaras, thoughts, memory storage, and recalling of cognates, thus providing information as and when needed.

BLISS SHEATH

Then finally we have the anandamaya kosha, the sheath around the soul or causal body, associated with a yet finer level of consciousness. It is the sheath of happiness, joy and bliss, and its food is joy. This kosha is beyond knowledge and experience, beyond the mind. It is about 'being', where we are bliss.

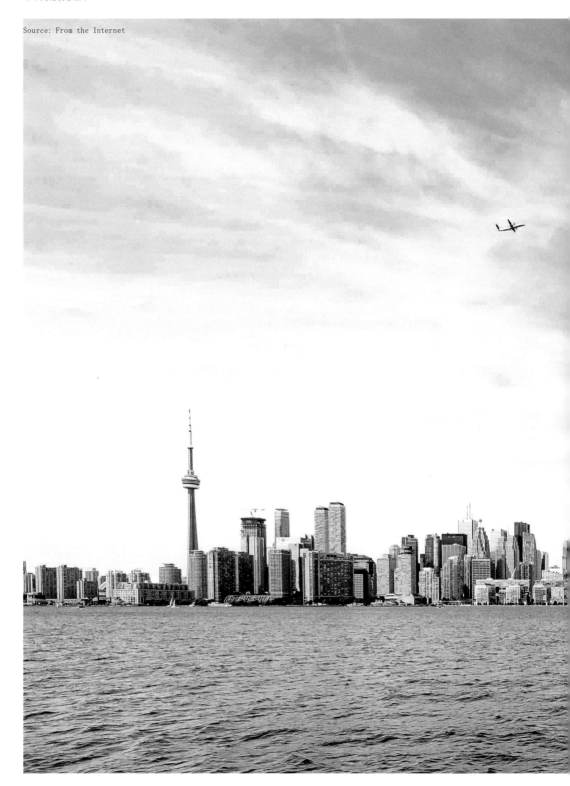

It is the subtlest of the five sheaths. On our journey we come across various spiritual stages offering us various levels of experiences, exposing our consciousness to more and more. We express joy at the level of the other four sheaths depending upon the resonance arising from the anandamaya kosha. Even this fifth kosha is not the end of the journey, although sat-chit-anand is considered to be such a high state.

During the spiritual journey all these sheaths are transcended. And this transcendence is another way of describing the journey of human evolution, the expansion of consciousness.

All the koshas have their inherent limitations, however subtle they may be. They are all interwoven, in fact, and not like the wooden Russian matryoshka dolls, one inside the next in a strictly sequential fashion. During meditation, we often have thoughts. Based on the kinds of thoughts we have, we can deduce the koshas where we are more or less restricted.

So regarding the aligment between the subtle bodies and koshas, we can say that:

• Ahankar, ego, is the subtle body of willpower and vitality, and is most closely associated with the pranamaya kosha.

• Manas, the thinking mind, is most closely associate with the manomaya kosha.

• And buddhi, intellect, is most closely associated with the vignanamaya kosha, the wisdom sheath.

What about chit, consciousness? Remember that consciousness is the canvas upon which the other three subtle bodies play out their functions, so it is associated with all three koshas of the subtle bodies

– pranayama, manomaya and vignanamaya. But consciousness is also there in every organ and every cell of the physical body, and at the other end of the spectrum it is also closest to the soul. So where is it?

Consciousness is everywhere. In a fully realized Yogi, consciousness is a 360-degree affair, flowing wherever it is needed in the moment. Consciousness spans all the koshas of the human being.

Even if we are not fully realized, and not aware of the full reach of our consciousness, that is only because we have not yet expanded it across the full spectrum of subconsciousness and superconsciousness. The koshas are another way to describe this spectrum of consciousness that we expand into as we go further and further on our journey.

Yoga is for this – a set of practices that refine our energy centers or chakras, refine the sheaths or koshas, and help us traverse through the various levels of consciousness.

Each one of us displays a consciousness based on its play within the complex web of these five sheaths, which are purified through the practice of meditation and cleaning. This purifying process is greatly accelerated by pranahuti. When we are able to harmonize our consciousness across all the five sheaths, we will see joy in life flowering on its own.

生命之生命
Life in Life

葛木雷什·D.巴特尔探讨了意识进化一个不同的方面。他描述了爱、慧能传递以及过程中连接和融合的需要。

世界上大多数人最想要的是什么?

如果调查一下对于这个问题的研究,你会找到一些答案,包括幸福、和平、信任、欣赏、自由、金钱等,但最根本的是爱。爱是生命的中心。大多数诗歌都是以爱的名义创作的,大多数音乐、艺术和电影亦如是。"上天是爱""爱是无敌"等等。所有伟大的神秘主义导师都在颂扬爱的重要性。所有伟大的圣人都爱上天、爱人类。佛陀并没有谈到爱,但他最著名的一句宣言是,他会一次又一次地轮回,直到每个人都得到解脱。难道这不是爱吗?

在下文中,我们关注意识和其他细体的进化,这是灵修的结果。那么,爱如何进入灵性科学这个领域之中呢?

首先要理解,因为事实上只有爱才能推动我们到达这个意识扩展之旅的终点,伴随着所有波折起伏。当然,如果没有爱也可以走过其中一段路,只要想获得个人的成长,但即便如此,你也要有足够的兴趣来面对这个过程。但是要达到静止的状态,要达到我们存在的中心,爱是必不可少的。爱令道路平坦。

让我们举一个世俗的类比——婚姻。在一段婚姻中对于另一半没有感情、没有爱，这会发生什么？如果没有爱，在亲密关系中能够轻易接受另一个人的小缺点、可笑的习惯吗？相反，当我们相爱时会发生什么？即便是另一个人的缺点都似乎如此可爱。当心中有爱的时候，我们更能接受。这会使道路平坦。爱能轻易克服障碍。

在婚姻或合作关系中，爱带来连接，最终是交融和合一。我们真诚地关心他人的安康。我们会把他们放在第一位，关心他们的感受、关心他们发生了什么，并以各种方式支持他们。我们感受到他们的感受，了解他们的想法。我们能够即刻说出彼此想说的话，回应对方的需求。你可能见过已经共同生活了一辈子的老夫妻，他们是如此紧密地结合，以至于完全不说话都能彼此理解。

照片来源于网络

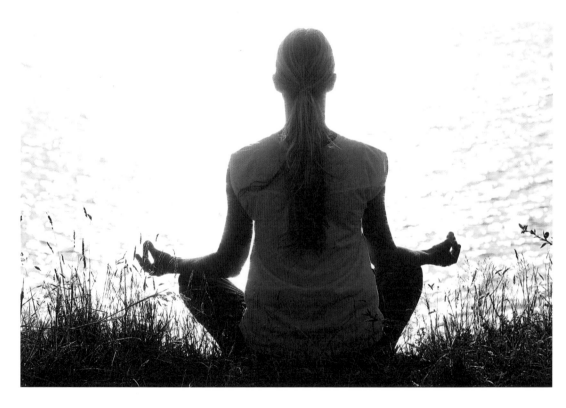

在母亲身上，连接和融合就达到了一个更加深刻的状态；付出的感觉定义了母亲和她的孩子的关系。付出是母性的精髓。母亲对于孩子并没有任何牺牲——无论是分娩、熬夜照顾生病的孩子或者去爱叛逆、不听话的孩子。对母亲来说，爱是其天性。

爱是连接。爱制造同情、悲悯，以及在最深层次上"感觉"到他人需要的觉知。在这些时刻，我们的一切都从我们的心流入他人的心，自然而然，不需要我们做任何事情。

我们不需要去到很远才知道爱打开了我们的心。即使在最人性化的层面，坠入爱河的经历，或是你对自己新生儿的爱，都会让你立即理解。世界展现瑰丽光彩，我们散发出一种很容易辨认的振动。

心有一种很有趣的特性——在其最纯净的状态中，实际上它是一个具有潜力的无限宇宙。通过灵性修习，它越来越向深层次开放，我们越来越扩展其存在的范围——意识谱，那么我们就越来越能够意识到自己与他人的心相连接。一颗纯洁的心能感觉到与其他每一颗心的连接。爱可以在心中产生真空，从而产生一种由心至心的流动。

现在让我们把这一点与扩展意识的灵性旅程联系起来。如果我们的修习是机械的、重复的和枯燥的，这会怎么样呢？你可以把它比作一段枯燥、没有爱的关系。没有火花、没有兴趣，因为没有融合，所以没有扩展。相反会有阻力，而修习变成了从自我出发，就如没有爱情的关系都是从自我出发的。当有兴趣的时候，心灵静修就会变得鲜活，并且每一刻都有奇迹、体验、开放和魔力。

如今，我们获得巨大的支持能够在心灵静修中培养这种兴趣。如何做? 在瑜伽慧能传递的帮助下进行。

慧能传递是最崇高、最精妙的爱。慧能源于本源,所以它可能是最纯粹的爱。当心向爱开放,慧能的涌流从内部滋养着我们,就像母亲的爱滋养着孩子。虽然慧能本身没有任何属性,它却溶解了边界,消除了分离。它将最粗重的形式变为最精妙的状态。它使我们纠缠的存在结节松动,为快乐和幸福规整出道路。慧能是终极的催化剂。

慧能从何而来,这种强烈的爱,源自我们存在的核心。慧能一直在那儿,在其本质和运用上都是无限的。它就存在于存在的构造之中,作为从本源传递出来的无力之力。

但知道它在那里是一方面;而另一方面是,能够利用慧能来进行意识的扩展,以及他人灵性的进化。这需要与本源有种特殊连接。这是一个师父的真正作用,一个最高修为的灵性向导。因为这样的大师能向我们的心传递精妙的本质,让意识随着真正的爱的纯洁而扩展。

师父像母亲一样,让我们出生到一个更高维度的存在,用传递理解的爱来充实我们。也许这就是辨喜大师所说的:"师父是上天为了走向我们所戴上的明亮的面具,随着我们不断地关注,面具也在逐步地脱落,而上天由此显现。"

有了慧能,生命就有了生命。心,是意识的画布,思维的细体在其上玩耍、被滋养。我们茁壮成长,我们绽放出花朵,最终我们的意识扩展达到其最完全的潜力、完全的合一。因此,我们的生命有了一种意义,否则,那只能在梦中找到。

Kamlesh D. Patel explores a different facet of the evolution of consciousness. He writes of love, transmission and the need for connection and communion along the way.

What do most people want more than anything else in the world?

If you examine the research about this question, you will find a number of answers, including happiness, peace, trust, appreciation, freedom, money, etc., but the most fundamental of all is love. Love is the center of life. Most poetry is created in the name of love, most music, art and film. "God is love" "Love conquers all" and so on. All great mystical teachers have extolled the importance of love. All the great saints have loved God and loved humanity. The Buddha did not speak about love, but one of his most famous statements is that he would keep coming back again and again until every human being is liberated. Is this not love?

In this series we have focused on the evolution of consciousness and the other subtle bodies, as a result of doing a spiritual practice. So how does love enter into this domain of the science of spirituality?

It is vital to understand, because in fact it is only love that can propel us to the end of this journey of expansion of consciousness, with all its ups and downs. Of course it is possible to go part of the way without love, just by wanting to grow individually, and even for that you need enough interest to commit to the process. But to reach that state of stillness, the center of our being, love is essential. Love makes the path smooth.

Let's take a worldly analogy. Marriage. What happens in a marriage where there is no feeling, no love for the other? Is it easy to accept the foibles and funny habits of another person at close quarters if there is no love? In contrast, what happens when we love? Even the faults of the other person seem so adorable. We accept so much more when love is there. It softens the way forward. Love overcomes obstacles with ease.

In a marriage or partnership, love brings connection and eventually communion and oneness. We are genuinely interested in the well-being of the other person. We put them first, we care about how they are feeling, what happens to them, and support them in all ways. We feel their feelings and know their thoughts. We finish each other's sentences and respond to each other's needs instantaneously. You have probably seen elderly couples who have been together a lifetime, who are so merged together that they understand each other completely without saying a word.

With motherhood, the state of connection and communion moves to an even more profound level; the feeling of giving defines a mother's relationship with her children. Giving is the quintessence of motherhood. Mothers do not sacrifice anything for their children – whether it be giving birth, staying up all night with a sick child or loving a rebellious, disobedient teenager. It is

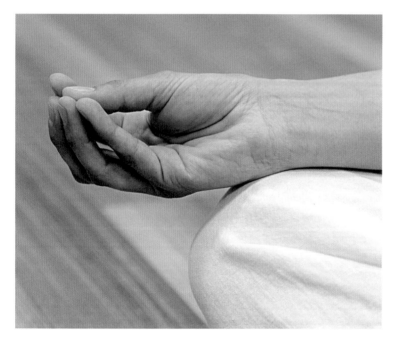

Source: From the Internet

natural for a mother to love.

Loving is connection. Love creates empathy, compassion, and the awareness to "feel" the other person's needs at the deepest level. At such moments, everything we have flows from our heart into the heart of the other, naturally, without our needing to do anything.

We don't have to look far to know that love opens our hearts. Even at the most human level, the experience of falling in love, or loving your newborn child, is instantly understood. The world appears rosy, and we exude a vibrancy that is easily recognizable.

The heart has a very interesting property – in its purest state it is actually an infinite universe of potentiality. The more it opens to deeper levels through a spiritual practice, the more we expand its field of existence, the spectrum of consciousness, and the more we become aware of our connection with the hearts of others. A pure heart feels connection with every other heart. A vacuum can be created in the heart by love, which results in a flow of current from heart to heart.

So let's relate this now to the spiritual journey of expanding consciousness. What happens if the practice we do is mechanical, routine and dry? You could compare it to a dry, loveless relationship. There is no spark, no interest, because there is no communion. So there is no expansion. Instead, there is resistance, and the practice is ego-driven, just like a loveless relationship is ego- driven. When interest is there, a spiritual practice comes alive and there is wonder, experience, opening and magic in every moment.

We are given enormous support to develop this interest in our spiritual practice in today's world. How? With the help of Yogic Transmission.

Transmission is the most sublime, subtle love. Transmission is from the Source, so it is the purest love possible. As the heart opens to love, the flow of

Transmission nourishes us from the inside, like a mother's love nourishes a child. While Transmission itself has no qualities, it dissolves boundaries and removes separation. It transmutes the grossest of forms to the subtlest of states. It loosens the knots of our entangled existence, making way for joy and bliss. Transmission is the ultimate catalyst.

Where does Transmission come from, this potent love that seeks out the very core of our being? Transmission is always there, and it is infinite in its nature and application. It is there in the fabric of existence as the subtlest forceless force emanating from the Source.

But knowing it is there is one thing; it is quite another thing to be able to utilize Transmission for the expansion of consciousness and spiritual evolution of others. That requires a special relationship with the Source itself. And that is the real role of a Guru, a spiritual Guide of the highest caliber. Because such a Guru can transmit that subtlest essence into our hearts, so that consciousness expands with the purity of true love.

Source: From the Internet

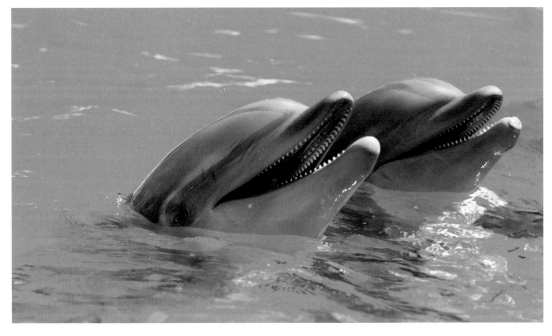

The Guru is like a mother, giving us birth into a higher dimension of existence, and filling us with a love that passes understanding. Perhaps this is what Swami Vivekananda meant by saying, "The Guru is the bright mask which God wears in order to come to us. As we look steadily on, gradually the mask falls off and God is revealed."

With Transmission, there is life in life. The heart, the canvas of consciousness upon which the subtle bodies of the mind play, is nourished. We thrive, we blossom, and eventually our consciousness expands to its fullest potential of complete Oneness. And thus our life takes on a meaning that is otherwise only found in dreams.

品格与生活方式
Character and Lifestyle

纯洁

在我心中纯洁等于神性。真理的本质便是纯洁。

关于上天我们能说些什么呢？神性是无限的。关于有限的议题我们可以写书。关于无限，恐怕只字不能出口。每当有人问上天是什么的时候，他们总是回答"神就是神"，多说一句都会显得十分幼稚。

意图的纯洁

有一次我与一位智者在一起，那是年底冬天的一个早晨。他独自一个人在那里，而我坐在一个角落。他伸出手指说"过来"。我就过去坐在他旁边。他在手背画了一条线，由于是冬天早上，指甲流下了一条白线。那时我在想，他到底在做什么。他说："这是一条运河。""是条运河。"只是想象那种。然后，从那条运河，他又用手指画了一条线，"你明白吗？"我问："明白什么啊？""五成的力量没有了。"接着他又画了一条线，第三条运河出现了。"这下你可明白了？"我说："明白了。"

那么让我们举一个日常生活的例子来说明这位智者的意思。你们手机上面有多少个应用？如果打开所有应用程序，电池很快就没电了。像我这样的人几乎没有什么

应用 (我有电话，但平时都处于关闭状态)，电池不会那么快没电。在生活当中，如果习惯于运行太多应用，有一个真正的来电你不会满意。一个女朋友不够，要众多女朋友，众多男朋友，好几辆汽车或摩托车。一切都要众多。但生活只有一个应用、一个目的，便可以通过最大限度地善用资源而让我们走得更远。

当我的目光锁定在了悟真理与上天时，我可能在踢足球，可能在开车，可能在经营业务，但我主要关注的对象始终是了悟真理与上天。我的意识全方面沉浸在那里，可以略为兼顾其他事物，但都只是为了支持这个主要的目标。

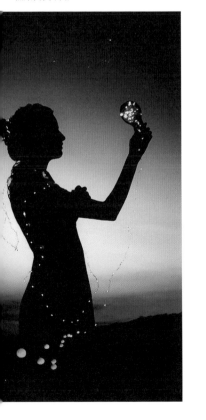

假如大家没有钱来马纳巴坎静修院，或许只好错过这次研讨会。那么很多人把金钱当作敌人，但事实并非如此。金钱如其他一切事物一样，关键在于如何使用。你的目的是什么？通过这种投入，你究竟想得到什么？我能买票来马纳巴坎，仅此而已。买衣服来遮体，别无他用。好了，能有个房子，但房子只有一个目的。不论住在哪里，有一套房子或是两套房子，或者是探望父母及孩子，不论如何目光始终锁定在了悟真理与上天。

如果思维有这种清晰度，那么道路会比较顺畅。在无限的海洋中你将一帆风顺。这是因为你有正确的理解。

风浪来来去去，但你理解："我不必担心这些，我有个保护者。有人在指导我，有人在等我。且说是心灵上的师父在指导，就这样。"命运就是这样塑造的。但需要有这种意图的纯洁。因此正视目标的纯洁、方法的纯洁、内在的纯洁以及态度上的纯洁能帮助我。

生活方式的纯洁

随着我们的进化，我们食用的饭菜、衣着打扮以及与生俱来的习惯需要逐渐适应自己的进化程度。你不可能漂浮在第十三点或心灵成长的顶点而依然在"谈恋爱"。但有人会问我："哦，原来这个也有可能？那么他的师父怎么让他走得那么远？"那是他的仁慈。假如让你体验第十三点，亦即最后一点的环境，你会否愿意呢？你们都迫不及待，但能在那里待多久？

一名乞丐呆在宫殿中，只能有赖于主人或君主的仁慈。要想能够呆下去，需要变得和君主一样。

因此，我们不仅要在内在实现进化，还要在自己的言谈举止以及生活方式上进化。需要来一个全方面的转变，一切都必须改变。

照片来源于网络

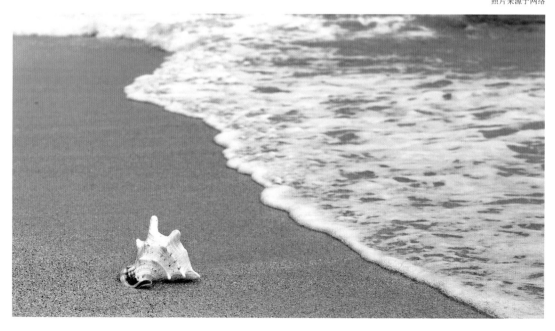

纯洁与非纯洁

已建立起来的宁静不应受到损害。

已建立起来的纯洁不应受到损害。

如何才能知道内在纯洁被污损了呢? 有哪些迹象可以说明? 几日前, 我读了一本很美的书:"有纯洁的良心, 兔子都能表现得和狮子一样, 而良心遭到损害后(充满不纯洁的良心)连狮子都会变得和兔子一样。"那么污损所带来的影响由此可见一斑。

我们现在谈的不是身体或灵魂的纯洁。不论身体多么纯洁、干净、闪闪发光、白皙无瑕, 难道能随你而到光明界吗? 身体无法进化, 有其自身的局限性。那么灵魂的纯洁呢? 其本质便是纯洁, 因此灵魂不可能不纯洁。进化的道路不会改变我们的身体, 也不会改变我们的灵魂。好了, 那我们究竟在谈什么呢? 是谈裹住灵魂的细体。其中, 主要是意识与心。此二者能让灵魂轻盈。

当你们向自己的父亲或母亲撒谎时, 你们的心会出现某种情况, 不是吗? 不要装圣人。告诉我, 你们一定撒过很多次谎。那时你们的心会发生什么呢? 如果去研究自己的心, 你们会发现自己在做不该做的事情时, 心跳会加速。纯洁受损的另一个症状是心变得沉重。然后会带来什么呢? 内疚与后悔。你会开始不喜欢自己,"我怎么能这样对自己的父母?"

这样一来会怎么样呢? 我的心本应轻盈, 有喜悦、有信心、有勇气去面对自己的父母, 因为我们没有做什么傻事。不论有意无意, 我都不应该出现任何污损。很多人会说:"对不起，我不是故意的，我没有想到这个人会是这样。爸爸，我很后悔。"不要欺骗父亲，也不要欺骗自己。你在污损心的纯洁。尽管身体的杂质和不净定然在人间埋葬或火化，但其振动会流入其他层面。我们应当十分小心。

欲念与幸福

我们的祈愿词道出了一个根本的事实："我们依然是欲望的奴隶……"直到还有这些欲念和欲望，它们将阻碍我们向前。

德国哲学家叔本华（Schopenhauer）曾提出这样一个问题："如何确定一个人开心或不开心？"他将开心定义为所有欲念得到满足。因此，用数学公式可以将一个人的幸福理解为：

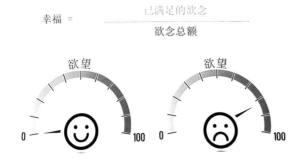

因此如果有十个欲念，假如其中有五个得到满足，你将有百分之五十的幸福。如果十个都得到满足，则化为百分百的幸福。欲念越多，满足所有欲念变得越难，幸福也就越少。因此，幸福与欲念总额成反比。

当我们完全没有欲念的时候会怎么样？

如果你的欲念总数为零，你的幸福将无极限。

在这个没有欲念的状态中我们不期待任何东西。当没有期待的时候我们也不会与自己以及他人玩游戏。由于自己对任何人没有任何期望，我们也不会操纵别人。

我们如何破坏自己内在的状态和人性呢？

这在《薄伽梵歌》第二章中提及，当欲念没有得到满足的时候，人会失望。失望导致愤怒，愤怒使平衡被打破；一旦失去了平衡，精神的平静就被打破，我们这就走向毁灭，我们的人性也随之而去。这就是为什么在自然之道中我们如此关注祈愿词的第二句："我们依然是欲望的奴隶，阻碍着自己的进步。"面对欲望要小心谨慎。

沙杰汗布尔的罗摩·昌德拉提出："越来越多的越来越少。"他这是在说什么呢？

他是指欲念：越来越多地有越来越少的欲念。当我们从数学的角度去看时，会发现这个简单的说法背后蕴含着莫大的智慧。如想要无限的幸福、无限的极乐，那么请减少自己的欲念，从越来越多到越来越少，最终化为零！学会安于自己。"上天啊，不论你给了我什么，将来又会给我些什么，我都很开心。"这难道意味着不能拥有那部iPhone手机？请自己想想。

我们的幸福究竟何在？心灵的满足感何在？

我们需要认识的是欲念只会增加不快乐，而零欲望则能无限增加幸福感。在这个状态当中，我们没有任何期盼，不会与自己或他人玩游戏，不会操纵人或对他们有任何期待。操纵人正是因为对其有所期待。

不论我们做些什么或想些什么，甚或有心愿起作用，都会

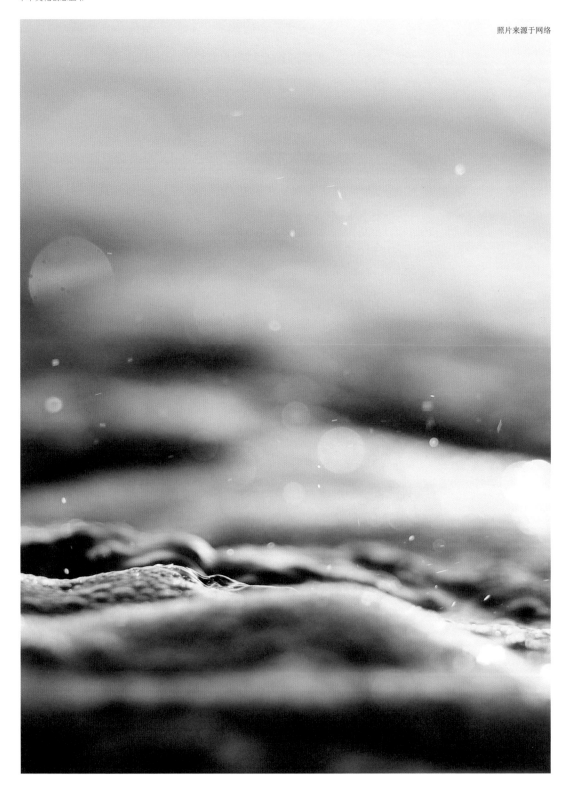

有两种后果。结果要么可喜，要么不可喜。当结果可喜时，我们心中会有平静，而后没有焦虑。当行动有利如期结果时，我们处于绝对平静的状态。当结果不如意时我们会感到不安。如某种行动不断产生良好结果，人就会有良好的心情。相反的轨道会如何呢？一次接一次的失望？也许不是一直出现不如意的事，但比如说某一个人一生都令人失望。那么这个人会使其不安，我们就不会再信任这种人。

欲念源自心。当妥当处理这些事情或一切顺利时，我们感到十分安详。当相反的情况出现时，我们就陷入不安。这些东西都会蒸发并产生新的印痕，波及第二轮点。这也是为什么第二轮点充满平静。每当来到第二轮点时，我们感到如此的平静以至于无心做俗世的任何事情。如果你是个商人，或学生、家庭主妇、丈夫，有一段时间你会对一切失去兴趣，这主要是因为这种宁静如此宜人，你完全不想被打扰，不想离开这个位置，这便是第二轮点的特征。

再来看看另一种情景。当有一个不断收获平静的来源时，会发生什么呢？

我们会爱上那个来源。又或者这种来源不断背叛我们，我们就会开始不喜欢它。而这种不喜欢就会蒸发到第三轮点，这里爱与恨始终存在。这便是第三轮点的特征。当有那么多的爱或恨时，便会蒸发到下一个轮点去制造很多的恐惧或勇气，这些便是第四轮点的特征。这就把我们带到下个点。当有过多的恐惧时，我们会开始在心中制造幻想，这会波及自己的意区，而意区不能容忍量幻想。

当精神受到如此大的干扰时，我们会失去自己的人性、自己作为人的特质。因此不应屈从这些事情，而要尽力去克服，否则会损害了自己整个生存。

愧疚

当我们坐在导师或师父面前时，基于欲念的思想，尤其是愧疚立马就会浮出表面。举例说明，一个容器中有浑浊的水，其中最重的东西都会往下沉。愧疚是我们身上所有印记当中最为沉重的印记，就好像铅一样，不断缠绕着我们。

很多时候愧疚是因为做了不该做的事情。但愧疚也有可能是因为没有做该做的事情。不是只有行为带来印记，没有及时行动也能制造致命的印记；比起某种行为带来的印记，这些要糟糕得多。失去的机会往往会缠绕着我们。"假如那一晚我温习多一点，知道正确答案的话，或许能获得八十五分而不是八十分的成绩。我就有资格被学院录取，我的前途就会……直到现在我还会做梦，梦见我在去学校考试的路上，然后想着铅笔在哪儿？"

很多时候，我们临睡时想到的首先是自己没有做好或完全没有去做的事。有时甚至会半夜惊醒："哟，我忘了签那份合约！"那些没有处理好的事情会制造极为不好的印痕并化为内疚，而这种内疚就会沉入底部。那些由于没有行动和蓄意做的事情会产生我们的系统中最为沉重的印记。这些印记无疑能清理，但需要较高级别的投入。在每个层面上都需要我们配合。

要自然，不需要有意识地揭露一切去说："请吧，请让一切出来。"不，我们不需要这样。自然即可。

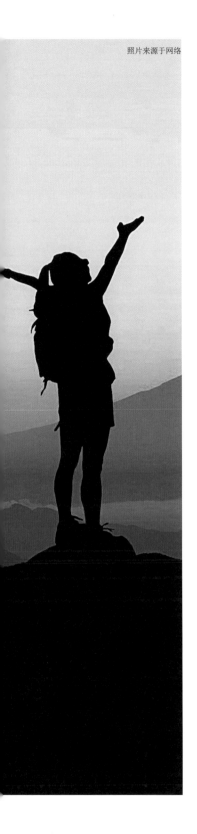

照片来源于网络

愤怒

大家都说愤怒是件坏事。但只有向外投射，才变得不好，比如朝向自己的亲朋好友或宠物等。愤怒的对象只能是自己，要说："哦，我居然有这种行为，多么愚蠢！我再也不应该如此。"警告自己，临睡时决心不再犯。甚至需要的话可以哭一下，向上天祈求原谅，誓不再犯。

这便是善用愤怒，不是向外投射而是朝向自己，促使自己改变。

激情

你没有自由任意暴露自己的激情，其存在是为了种类的生存，仅此而已。这种激情不可能毁灭。

自我与卓越

不论我们做些什么，我们必须卓越，这一点与自负无关。当我们绘画时，有无达到卓越？读书时有没有优异的成绩？人们说："我不会优秀，我要做谦卑不自大的人。"不必自大，但不能以卓越为代价。生命的目标是这个：不论做什么，我们必须卓越。卓越！人们会说："但是这样我的小我就会膨胀。"什么情况下小我会膨胀呢，我不停地说："看我的工作多么美妙，是我做的，你可做不到。"我不能用来伤害别人而是不断将手指转向自己："好了，我的确可以比上次做得好一点。"自我不可毁灭。人们说："我要毁掉小我，摆脱小我的影响。"这是不可能的。

真正的自我不会与他人比较，只会将自己与昔日的表现比较。这样的话自我可以起到建设性的作用，否则可能引发灾难。

面对自己的老板时，你知道可以欺骗他，但你无法欺骗自己。当你欺骗你的老板时，实际上你在丧失自己的潜力，在牵制自己的潜力。有时候你的老板叫你"跳"，你应该能够去问他"多高"? 不论做什么，要做到卓越。冥想的时候，我应该冥想达到卓越。工作的时候，我应该工作达到卓越。不仅在工作上卓越，在处理其他事情的时候也要卓越，其他事情也同等重要。而其中最重要的是我与生命的本源那种柔软而充满爱的连接。

一体化

如何去除生活中不必要的事物?

专心致志。曾经有人对我说："爱赚多少钱就赚多少钱，但花钱要有智慧。"但如果懂得花钱的智慧，为何还会需要那么多呢?

我们应该明白，努力挣钱去维持物质生活其实是为了支持心灵静修上的努力。这两个翅膀——精神与物质必须同时飞翔，必须一体化。我不是说要去平衡二者。我喜欢用"一体化"去形容。我们应该能够将灵性的翅膀伸入自己的物质生活。当我做生意的时候，如果手段正当纯洁，赚十亿或百亿元又有什么分别? 这样我就不会有后悔的事情。不论做些什么，心中无愧就可以了。如有必要，我甚至可以转让，这会让我的心也打开。不是说我挣钱只为了家人或自己。有能力的话，大可以进一步探索。

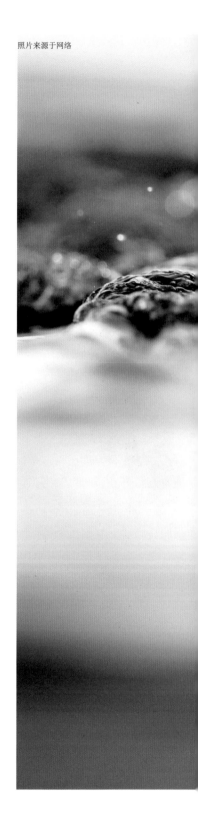

照片来源于网络

谦卑

我们谈过纯洁是如何编织命运的，但我们并没有谈到不洁是如何毁灭我们的命运。请自己想一想：有哪些情绪能破坏我的纯洁？发脾气是第一，对吧？憎恨是另一个。还有哪些呢？怀疑、诱惑、恐惧、愧疚、懒惰、自大、妒忌、比较、偏见等都只代表小部分。所以需要小心。现在你们已经认清了自己的敌人。懒惰——是，无知的话，恐怕很难。无知的人并不知道自己无知，那就是无知的另一面！因此，知道了自己的敌人有哪些之后，我们就可以在其到来前就认出。

纯洁编织命运

怀疑、诱惑、恐惧、愧疚、懒惰、自负、妒忌、比较、偏见、爱、耐心、包容、接受、信仰、纪律、谦卑。

再来看看有哪些好的东西可以延长，乃至深化我们的纯洁？能不能以这种方式认清自己的好友？爱是第一个。耐心——是，包容、接受、信仰、纪律——是，接受！有一堆好友。

在《薄伽梵歌》中，黑天神指出了二十一或二十二个必备的崇高品质以应对这种斗争。我不知道他为什么那么喜欢把人生比作战争。他说，应当将这个生命当作被自己居住的宫殿来保护，其围墙有这二十一或二十二个品质做城门。然后他说，这些城门都要用这些品质保护好。但后门是要害（没有人关注后门），敌人往往会从后门而入，攻其不备。然后他说，后门是用谦卑来守护。没有谦卑，其他所有的门都难以防守。

在十项格言中，在解说最后一项格言的结尾时，一位智者高度强调了谦卑与简朴的品质。他说，有了谦卑与简朴的品质，可以认为所需要的一切都有了，再也没有别的东西。心怀谦卑之人，非但有敬重，不必说出来的敬重，他们还颇有帝王的庄严。在外面时，这种人的言谈举止让他们如皇族那样鹤立鸡群。你们会清楚地觉得，他们好像是皇家出身，身上有一点不同。

在一个灵性的人当中，如有这种灵性的庄严或帝王般的品质，其言谈举止也会充分反映这一点。甚至在没有走动或说话时，也难以隐藏。谈吐恭敬、礼貌。在自然之道中，我们不仅希望有良好的沟通，还希望进而达到一种心灵的交流：从沟通到交流。

一切都要卓越，却不要唯我独尊。这种态度会毁了我们。直到我们还认为自己伟大时，我们将继续在自己周围建筑自大之墙，自绝于神性王国的其他一切。我们在囚禁自己并变得孤独。即使亲朋好友环绕左右，我们也会身陷孤独。

只有当我们打破自大之墙并将自己当作宇宙微不足道的仆从而臣服时，我们才会化为空无、征服自己各种倾向，这种生命着实快乐。这意味着全然归依。

有谁会心甘情愿归依？自我就在那里拦路。但你也可以宠一下自我，"我会在自己的归依中达到卓越"。这会帮助你并让你逐渐告别自我。

自然性

纯洁不需要说出来，爱不需要说出来。尽管只字未言，在不知不觉中，也能在心中留下印象。玫瑰花会不会提问我应不应该散发芬芳？尽管如此，我们的智力还是会问："我应该这样做还是那样做？"当我的内在本性是不断发出纯洁与爱的时候，何必限制自己说"好了，此时此刻我只做这个"？这样并不自然。这样的话我就变得和那些人造喷香机一样。大家见过喷香机吧？当我们经过那里的时候，这些喷香机会辨认出有人经过并喷出一股香味。

真实

如果我们继续伪装自己，不做真实的自己。甚至连与自己配偶的关系、亲朋好友的关系都无法维持。因为我们总是在撒谎，总是想炫耀。其实没有必要在意别人对你的印象，你究竟想愚弄谁？

做不真实的人需要很多的努力。撒谎需要努力，还要记住说了些什么。撒谎需要创意，但想说真话你就要简单。真话纯洁，直接发自我们的心。对于这种人，上天也会爱意倾盆。这种人满足于自己的简朴和纯洁，并不企图给人留下良好印象。这是因为他们知道自己是什么。智慧的瑜伽士们就是这样。他们不想给任何人留下什么印象。他们是什么就是什么。

苦恼

煤炭与钻石有何分别？都是碳。当煤炭经受了巨大压力并受热时会化为钻石。我们的生命也是如此，尽管知道最终结果一定很好，但我们却不愿意经受苦恼。童年的记忆，乃至现在的经历都会告诉你，我们无不喜欢谈起那些痛苦的经历。"我一直徒步到机场呢。"我们甚至引以为豪，而假如是坐车去的，恐怕就没有什么可骄傲的了。

当经历了困难时期并以正直的方式度过时，你可以说："我做到了！"困难时期的确让我们变得坚强。假如不需要考试，你们当中有谁愿意上课？或许只有少数，真正认真对待学业的人才会说："考试不考试，我还是要学习。"这种人是另一种类的人。但我们却害怕考验和考试。

假如让我们选择，就不愿意参加考试，对吧？这恰恰就是需要纠正的问题。生活也应该一样。人生充满考验，各种各样的考验，连大师们都不能幸免。这些考验不像考试那样考的只是你的能力，生活中遇到的挑战让我们为成就大业做好准备。

当生活中出现意外时，我们应该从那些时刻中学习而不应该与之相抗衡。应该学习，努力解决问题而非灰心丧气。如开始灰心，头脑就处于不安，那么内在的那个雷达、那个向导本身也会随之而不安，此时我们得不到来自内在的指导，无法做出正确的决定。因此，遇到挑战时，应当很好地保持警惕。与其抵抗不如邀请其前来。

这也是为什么我们不断强调："接受苦恼。"不接受的话，我们永远都无法理解其目的。这些苦恼本来可以为我们做什么？能带领我们达到什么境界？一旦我们拒绝生活中自己不

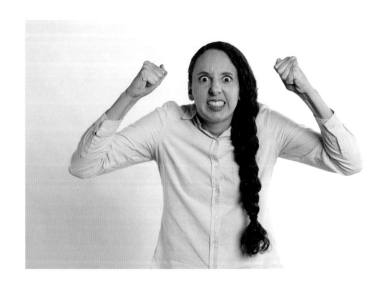

照片来源于网络

想要的东西时，这些经验教训就错过了。应当泰然处之，带着静默的心、勇敢的心，但需要很多的勇气。经历了某些情况之后，你会变得更加坚强。

如果不接受，什么也学不到。如只是一般接受，只能继续做一般的人。让我们带着喜悦，愉悦地接受这些苦恼，然后再看看会涌现出什么样的美景。

这需要很大的勇气和自信。这样你就能成功，你的事情也许失败，但在生命的考试中你已经及格了，而我们要的就是这一点。我们不像懦夫那样逃跑，而是面对生活，继续前进并以此来制造自己的命运。与那些躲避生活的人不同，我们带着勇气和信心面对生活。

经受人生的考验与苦难，无人能幸免。普通人与神性人的区别就在于此——他们能带着微笑经受一切，而我们却做不到。

"愉悦地接受，则苦难会起到应有的作用。"否则这些横竖都需经历的苦难不会起任何作用，我们也只是白白痛苦，却没有任何积极的成果出现。愉悦地接受，经受过程就能结出灵性成果。因此需要接受。

不断期待美好时光的人永远都找不到幸福。接受当下，与世界泰然相处，你这一生就安好。你已经掌握了自己的生命。

这下你可以带着信心从容不迫地走过人生风云却从不受影响；这里不受影响的意思是不吸收印记，自己没有，也不让他人产生印记。非但自己没有制造印记，也没有让他人制造印记。你的生存不再产生波纹。即便有，只是纯洁与爱的波纹。毕竟在他人身上制造印记也是一个问题。

紧迫性

不论需要做一些什么，不论能完成一点什么工作，趁尚有精力的时候尽快完成，尤其是最为重要的东西——领悟上天。你有时间去读书，有时间积累知识，有时间坐下来冥想并接收慧能及来自上面的恩典和祝福。等到一定的时候你会可望却不可及，你会说："哎哟，我这个疼痛啊"，躺在床上也得不到安宁！这种仰卧的状态如何坐下来冥想或接收慧能？实在很难，因为身体的问题始终会缠绕着你。因此，不论需要付出什么代价，让我们现在就去成就能够成就的一切，而不要把事情推迟到日后。

大家需要为自己设好目标，这些目标不用和别人分享，但一定要设好目标并确保自己能达到。迈向这些目标的每一小步都会让我们意志的力量变得越来越强。有时候人们会设定非常高的目标，请不要这么做。一步一步来——你的头脑能处理、你的心能接受的那种目标最好。生活可以有小目标，但应当始终不忘主要目标。所有这一切都应该把我带往至高。至高便是领悟上天，亦即合一。

睡眠

假如人们能在作息方面稍微有点规律，他们完全可以改变自己的一生。只需要调整一下生活，在以下两个方面养成规律：第一，睡得好；第二，晚上9点钟前睡觉。

请从作息开始入手。早一点睡觉，也许这个听起来很愚蠢，也许你们在心中会产生蝴蝶效应，带来严重的后果。大家

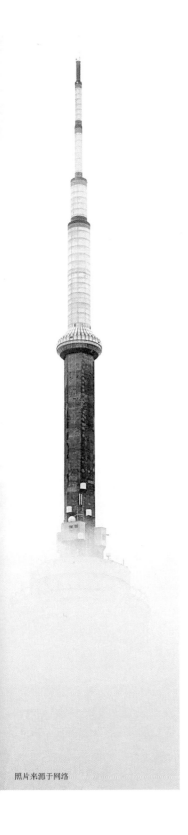

可曾听说过这个理论？南美洲亚马孙森林中有只蝴蝶鼓翼，导致一片叶子开始拍动，接着两片、三片叶子开始拍动，最终北美洲出现暴风雪。睡眠有一点规律，良好、深入的睡眠会决定大家一整天中的精神状态。

所以，这个选择在于你们。你们想过汹涌海洋般的生活吗，也就是现在最吸引人的那种生活？完全无法知道到底有什么事情在发生，在紊乱的意识浪潮中，你们将迷失自己。相反，当意识处于稳定状态时，哪怕小小的变化或不同都会十分明显。反过来说，海洋中那块可怜的岩石什么也不会发生。这就是为什么朋友那么投契，因为他们和这些海洋一样，吵来吵去也不会发生什么事。但是在有爱的关系中，哪怕你用稍微不同的眼神看对方就会起波纹。"哦，他今天用这种眼神看我。"这的确发人深思。

有句话很美，说你可以顺流而游，也可以逆流而上，但后者会消耗自己。

瑜伽经典十分重视左右两个鼻道。瑜伽经典中右鼻道被认为是阳脉（Pingala），左鼻道（Ida）则主导夜间的时间被认为是月脉。理想的情况是白天以右鼻道为主，夜晚则以左鼻道为主。为什么呢？我们恐怕没有时间去讨论为何以及如何，但是我们可以记住这一点，即我们的生理节奏受太阳及月亮运动的影响。当出现失调时呼吸鼻道会调换。

这也是为什么旧时人家会起来检查自己的呼吸，如果呼吸不正常，他们就会喝开水并进行诸如调息

（Pranayama）、散步等。如细心留意，在日出和日落时分，你们会发现从右到左或从左到右的缓慢轮替。而假如这个时候能坐下来冥想，我想告诉大家简直会跟火箭一样直线升空，因为此时交感神经体系与自主神经体系处于平衡状态。

那么睡得比较晚的人会发生什么呢？你们可以观察一下，当你们按时睡觉，比如晚上9点钟或10点钟时，请观察呼吸会从右鼻孔转向左鼻孔。如果获得足够的睡眠，早上一起床，右鼻孔就会自动开始主导。经过几千年，我们的生理体系发生了演化，让太阳升起刺激到一些荷尔蒙规律。如果顺着这个节奏，健康状况自然就会改善。如果逆着节奏，犹如逆流而游，会随着时间而消耗自己。当精力和青春的活力开始衰落时，你们就真的是逆流而上，而到时候你们的健康状况会说明很多问题，不如趁早形成良好节奏。

我想夜间活动是现代世界的一大诅咒。由于电力，现在昼夜不分，缺乏睡眠反映出种种不规律，你们的健康就会因此而受影响。由于神经系统开始衰竭，你们的免疫力也会随之而下降。

已有广泛的研究证明夜间工作对健康的影响，尤其是那些别无选择，不这样就会失业的人群。如果去观察他们的健康，我们会发现他们老得比较快。我们多数人并不需要上夜班。我们有选择，然而我们的生活方式却如那些无可奈何、只好通宵工作的人一样。我们自愿熬夜，观看着各种各样的东西。

因此不论从那个角度来看，灵性也好、健康也好，这种习惯只会带来不利于自己的结果。既然如此，何必冒险？做亏本生意有什么好处？所以，请大家早点睡觉，这真的会给你们带来很大帮助。

在古杰拉特语中有一种说法：早睡早起，身强思敏，财福常在。这些话很有智慧。

只有健康的身体能有健康的思维，反之亦然。很多人会辩论说有健康的思维带来健康的身体，但身体不健康，思维也会紊乱。"唉，我的腿不行了，我的手不行了，而且还有那么多不行。"然后你们就拼命地看病吃药。开始担心，心自然就乱了。这下何谈编织命运？仅仅因为没有尊重自然的节奏，你已经选择了毁灭的道路。

照片：沈文成摄

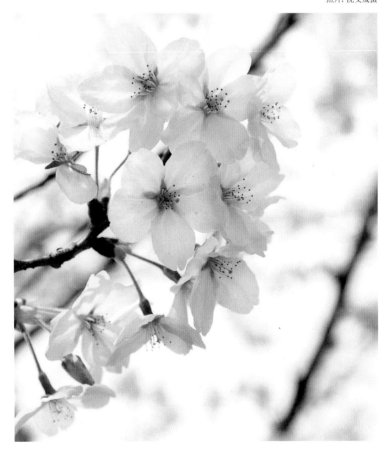

有一项格言说要与大自然和谐一致，抵抗恐怕得不到任何好处。有句话很美，说你可以顺流而游，也可以逆流而上，但后者会消耗自己。晨间大自然的能量流向本源的方向，这并不是一种物质能量。我们最好与这种能量一致。就像我昨天说的，由于不够强壮，只要稍微有一点"剂量"，你们就被击倒了。

所以如想更上一层楼，不论如何，你们都必须调整睡眠。否则这一生都会花在这种挣扎之中。起床时颓废、没有睡好，冥想就难免变得很难。无法正确冥想，也就没有正确的灵性状态。这下没了正确的意识去处理哪怕俗世的事情。你已经把指导力量——意识——连根拔起，让自己受到那么多东西的影响。这下自己变得脆弱。人就越来越像收垃圾的，成天积累印记，整个人陷入恶性循环。

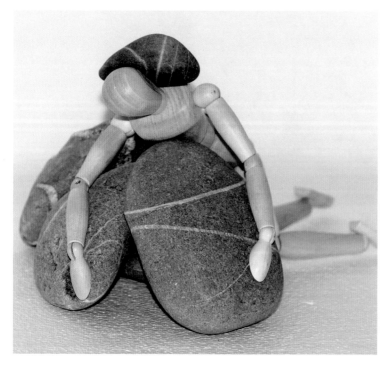

照片来源于网络

相反，如果有良好的状态、纯洁的状态、喜悦的状态，我们就会更加感恩。这种发自内心的感恩会在我们的创造者和自己之间建立联系纽带。这种纽带会极大地惠及我们，而受益越多，越会想做得越来越多。

Purity

To my heart, purity is akin to God. The essence of Reality is purity.

What can be said about god? He is infinite. On limited subjects we can write books, on the subject of infinity, we cannot even speak one word. Whenever someone asked what god is, they always replied, "he is what he is!" it would be childish to describe anything further.

Purity of Intention

Once I was sitting with a wise man. It was a wintery morning in November or December. He was alone and I was seated in one corner. He pointed a finger and said, "Aao [come]." So I went and sat nearby and he made a line on his hand like this and it made a mark because it was a winter morning. If you scratch yourself it will make a white line. I was wondering what he was doing. He said, "This is a water canal." "Yes, this is a water canal." It was a make - believe type of thing. Then, from the same canal, he scratched himself and drew another line. "You understand?" I said, "What" "Fifty percent of the power is reduced." Then he scratched himself again. A third canal. "Now do you understand?" I said, "Yes."

Now let us take an everyday example to elucidate

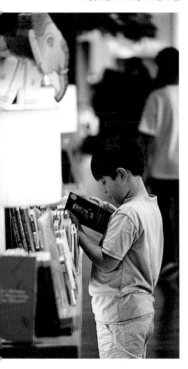

the wise man's point how many applications do you have on your phones? If you leave them all running, all open, the battery drains very quickly. For a person like me with almost no applications (I have a phone that usually remains switched off anyway), the battery won't drain so quickly. In life, if you get used to running too many applications, you are not happy with one true caller. One girlfriend is not enough you want multiple girlfriends, multiple boyfriends, multiple cars, or multiple scooters. Everything you want in multitudes. But having one application in life, one goal in life, will take us somewhere through an optimum utilisation of our inner resources.

Having one application in life, one goal in lite will take us somewhere through an optimum utilisation of our inner resources.

When my focus is God Realisation, I can be playing soccer, I can be driving, I can be running a business, but my main focus remains God Realisation. My consciousness is fully drenched there. It is allowed to attend to other things very minimally, and I do other things only to support this main endeavor.

If you didn't have money to come to Manapakkam, you would have missed out on this seminar. So many people consider money as an enemy, but it is not. Money is like any other thing - it is how you use it. What is the goal? What do you want to achieve by that investment? I buy my tickets to come to Manapakkam. That's all. I buy clothes so that I can be protected. There is nothing more than that. I have a house. So be it, have a house, but it is to serve one and only one purpose. Wherever I stay, whether I have one house or two houses or I'm visiting my father or mother or my children, whatever it is, my main focus is God realization.

If you have this clarity of mind, then you will make it through smoothly. Your sail will be smooth through the infinite ocean because you have the right understanding.

Storms may come and go, but you still have that greater understanding that, "I don't have to be worried about all these things. I have a protector. Somebody is guiding me. Someone is waiting for me. Master is guiding and that's that!" That is how we make our destiny you see. But I must achieve this purity of intention. So it is purity of goal, purity of method, purity within, and purity in my attitudes that will help me.

Purity of Lifestyle

As we evolve, the food that we take, the clothes that we wear, and all the habits that we are born with have slowly to be adjusted to our level of evolution. You can't float on the thirteenth point at the culmination of spiritual growth and still be dating. But then someone would ask me. "Oh, so that's possible? Then how did master allow him to get that far?" It is his mercy. Aren't you willing to experience the atmosphere of the thirteenth point, the last point you are all anxious to do so, but how long can you live there?

A beggar can't be in a palace for more time than the mercy of the lord or the mercy of the king allows. We have to become like a king to deserve to stay in the palace.

So we must evolve not just from within but in our manners and in our lifestyle. A complete turnaround is necessary. Everything must Change.

Purity and Impurity

Serenity once created should not be spoiled. Purity once created should not be spoiled. How will you know if your inner purity has been compromised? What are the signs? A few days back, I read in a beautiful book, "With a pure conscience, even a rabbit acts like a lion and with a compromised conscience (impurity-filled conscience), even a lion will behave like a rabbit." So this is just a hint of how we can perceive the compromised purity of the heart.

We are not talking at the moment about the purity of

the body or soul. However pure the body may be, washed, cleaned up - a gleaming, snow - white body - will it come with you to the Brighter World. The body cannot evolve. It has its limitations. What about the soul's purity? Purity is its nature. It cannot be impure. This evolutionary path is not going to change our body, nor will it change the soul. Fine, then what are we talking about? Which purity do we want to maintain here? It is the purity of the subtle bodies, which envelop the soul. Mainly, it is that of consciousness and of the heart. Thereby, the soul will be lightened.

When you lie to your father or to your mother, something happens to the heart, no? Don't try to be saintly. Tell me, you must have lied so many times. What happens to your heart at that time when you study the heart, you will find that if you do something wrong, your heart starts pumping fast. Another sign of compromised purity is that the heart becomes heavy. And then what takes over? Guilt and regret. You start disliking yourself. "How could I do such a thing to my parents?"

Now what happens? I should have had lightness in the heart, joy in the heart, confidence in the heart, and the courage to face my parents because I have not done anything stupid. I should not have compromised anything at any level, knowingly or unknowingly. Many people give the excuse, "Oh, sorry. I did it unknowingly. I didn't know that this person was like that. Papa, I am sorry I did this." Don't fool your father and don't fool yourself. You are compromising your purity of heart. Although the complexities and impurities of the body will be buried or burned here, their vibrations will go on into other dimensions. We have to be very careful .

Desire and Happiness

Our prayer says one fundamental thing: "We are yet but slaves of wishes..." As long as we have these desires and wishes, they will stop us from going further.

The German philosopher Schopenhauer asked the question, "How can we determine whether a man is happy or unhappy?" He defined true happiness as the complete satisfaction of all desires. You could say that the happiness of a person can be described mathematically as:

So if you have ten desires and five are fulfilled, you have fifty percent happiness. If ten are fulfilled, you have one hundred percent happiness. The more desires you have, the harder it will be to fulfil them all, and so the less happy you will be. Happiness is inversely related to numbers of desires.

What happens when you have no desires at all?

The denominator becomes zero. Anything you divide by zero is infinity. If you have zero desires, limitless will be your happiness.

In this desireless state, we don't expect anything. When we don't expect anything, we don't play games with ourselves and others. We don't manipulate others because we don't expect anything from anyone.

How do we destroy our inner condition and our humanness?

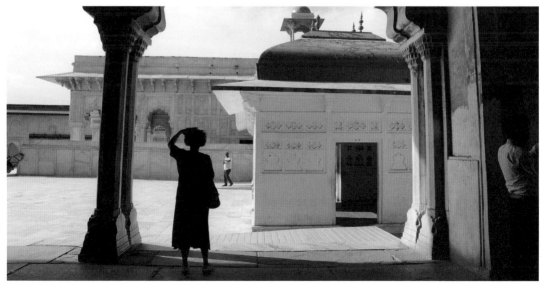

It is mentioned in the Bhagavad Gita, in chapter two, that when desires are not fulfilled there is disappointment. Disappointment leads to anger, anger makes us lose our balance, and once we lose our balance, our mental equilibrium, we are destroyed and lose our humanness. That is why in Sahaj Marg we pay so much attention to that second line of the prayer: "we are yet but slaves of wishes putting bar to our advancement." We have to be careful with those things.

Ram Chandra of Shahjahanpur spoke about. "More and more of less and less." What is he talking about?

He is talking of desires: more and more of less and less of desires. When you look at it in a mathematical way, you see so much wisdom in that simple statement. If you want to have infinite happiness, infinite bliss, then minimise your desires, from more and more to less and less and finally to zero! Make peace with yourself. "My lord, whatever you have given me and you continue giving me in the future, I am happy." Does that mean you should not have an iPhone? You think about it.

Where lies our happiness? Where is that contentment of the soul of the heart?

We have to realise that having desires is only going to increase our unhappiness and having zero desires is going to infinitely increase our happiness. In this state, we don't expect anything. When we don't expect anything, we don't play games with ourselves or with others. We don't manipulate others because we don't expect anything from them. We start manipulating people precisely when we have expectations from them.

Whatever we do, or even think, or even will through our heart, there are two consequences. Either the results are favourable or not favourable. When the results are favourable, we are at peace and we have no other anxiety afterwards. We are at absolute peace when our action is fulfilled as per our expectation. When the results of the actions are against us, we are disturbed. If one action gives good results and it keeps happening like this, a person develops a happy disposition. What happens to the other person who is on the other trajectory, where there is disappointment after disappointment? It may not be all the time, but let us say he has disappointment from only one person all the time in his life. That person creates disturbance in him, and he stops trusting that person.

Desires arise in the heart. When these things are handled properly and when things go right, you feel a lot of peace. When the opposite happens, you are disturbed. Both evaporate and form other impressions, affecting the second point. That is why the second point is full of peace. Whenever you reach that point you find so much peace that you don't feel like doing anything at all in the world. If you are a businessman or you are a student or a housewife or a husband, you lose interest in everything that you do for some time because this peace is so inviting. You don't want

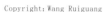

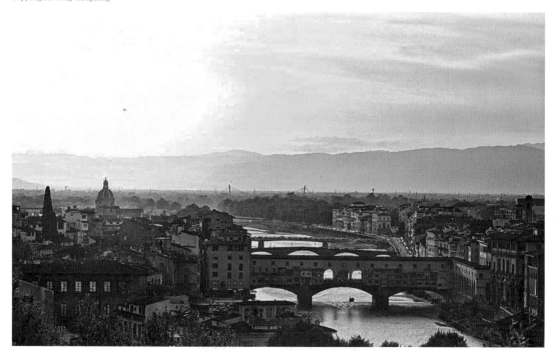

to be disturbed at all. You don't want to be distracted from this. That is the quality of the second point.

Now look at the other scenario. When there is a continuous harvest of peace from one source, what happens?

You fall in love with that source, or if it goes on betraying you all the time, you start disliking that thing. And that again gets evaporated to the third where hatred and love are perpetually present. It is the quality of the third point. Similarly, when there is so much love or its opposite, it evaporates to the next one, where it creates either a lot of fear or a lot of courage, and they are the qualities of the fourth point. This also gives rise to the next point. When you have too much fear, you start creating illusions in your mind and that affects your cosmic region. And the cosmic region (the mind) cannot tolerate illusions.

When the mind gets disturbed like that, you have lost your humanity, your human traits. So, we should not succumb to these things. We must overcome them as early as possible. Otherwise they spoil our entire existence .

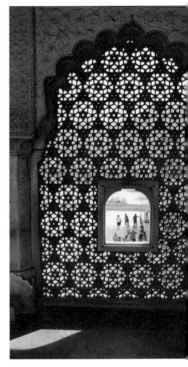

Copyright: Na Zemin

Guilt

When we are seated in front of a preceptor or in front of Master, thoughts that are based upon desires, especially on guilt, come immediately to the surface. Take the example of a container filled with muddy water, where the heaviest objects sink to the bottom. Guilt is the heaviest of all the samskaras that we carry. It is like lead and it bothers us so much.

Most of the time, guilt is a product of something that I should not have done and I did. Guilt can also be because of something I should have done but did not do. It is not only our actions that promote samskaras. Our inactions can create lethal samskaras that are worse than those created by our actions. Lost opportunities haunt us. "I had studied a little bit extra that night and given the correct answer, I would have received a mark of eighty - five percent instead of eighty percent. I would have been admitted to college. My career would have been..." I still get dreams at night where I am going to college for my exams and think, "where is my pencil? "

Most of the time, when we go to bed what comes to our mind first is the thing that we didn't do properly, or the things that we didn't do at all. Sometimes they wake you in the middle of the night. "I forgot to sign that contract!" Those things that we don't do properly create very bad impressions, and they become guilt, which stays at the rock bottom. Those samskaras created by inactions, deliberate inactions, amount to the heaviest of the samskaras in our

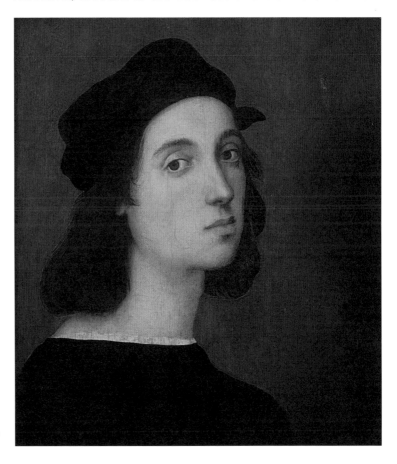

Raffaello Sanzio

system. They can be removed, no doubt, but then a commitment of a very high order is required. Your cooperation at every level required.

Be natural. You don't have to consciously expose everything, saying "please, please show it, please show it. " No, we don't want to do that, be natural.

Anger

Everybody says that anger is a bad thing. It is only bad if you project it outside, on your loved ones or on your dog perhaps. Anger should only ever be projected on yourself. You say, "Oh, I did this. How stupid of me! I should not do this again." Warn yourself. Resolve at bedtime. You can cry if you have to. Beg forgiveness from God: "My Lord, I will not do this again. This is it."

That is the right utilisation of anger, not projected outside, but projected towards oneself to change.

Passion

You don't have free licence to expose your passion. It is for the survival of your species. There is nothing more than that you see. It can never be destroyed.

Ego and Excellence

Whatever we do, we must excel and that has nothing to do with ego. When we paint, are we excelling in that when we study, are we excelling in our studies? People say, "I will not excel. I want to be humble and non egotistical." Don't have ego, but not at the cost of excelling. The purpose of life is this: we must excel in everything that we do. Excel! People say, "Oh, but my ego will go up." Ego will go up only when I repeatedly say, "Look at my work. It's so wonderful. I did it. You can't do it." Ego is not to be used to hurt others. It is to keep pointing the finger back towards myself saying, "OKAY, I can do it better

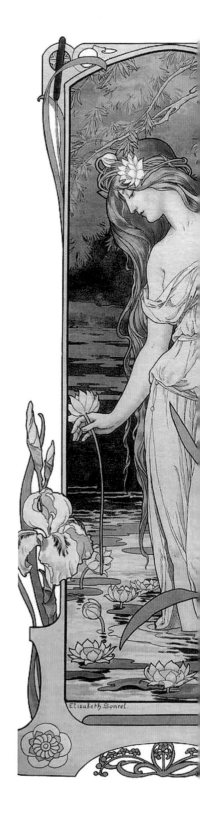

Elisabeth Sonrel.

than I did last time." Ego can never be destroyed. People say, "I want to annihilate it completely and remain ego-free." It is not going to happen.

With a true ego, I am not comparing myself with others. I am comparing myself with my previous performance. Then, the utilisation of the ego can be productive. Otherwise it can be disastrous.

With your boss, you know you can cheat him, but you cannot cheat yourself. When you cheat your boss, actually you are cheating your potential. You are putting a brake on your potential. Sometimes if the boss says "jump", you should be able to say "How high?", Excel in everything that you do. When I meditate I must excel. When I work I must excel, not only in the work but in how I look after other things also. Other things are no less important. And the main thing is my tender, loving connection with the origin of life.

Integration

How to remove unnecessary things in your life?

Remain focused on one and one thing only. Once someone told me, "Make as much money as you like but spend it wisely." But if you spend it wisely, why do you need so much?

We have to realise that our efforts to make money for the sake of our material life are only in support of our spiritual efforts. Both wings the spiritual as well as the material wing, must fly together, must be integrated. I am not trying to say that you must balance them. I like to use the word integrate. I must be able to extend the wings of spirituality into my material life. Then there is beauty in material proliferation. When I do business, how does it matter whether I am going from ten crores to one hundred crores, if the means that I apply are honest and pure? Then I will have no regrets. There will be no guilt for whatever I may do. If need be, I can transfer it, which will also open my heart. It is not that

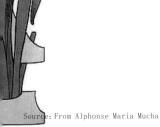

Source: From Alphonse Maria Mucha

I make money only for my loved ones or myself. If you have the ability, explore it further.

Humility

We have spoken about how purity weaves our destiny, but we have not talked much about the impurities that destroy our destiny. Think about it for yourselves what kinds of moods can destroy my purity? Anger is number one, right? Hatred is another one. What are the other ones? Doubt, temptation, fear, guilt, laziness, ego, jealousy, comparison and prejudice, to name a few. You have to be so careful. Now you have identified your enemies. Laziness - yes. With ignorance we can't do much. Ignorant people don't know they are ignorant. That's the other ignorant part of it! So knowing the enemies now, we can all recognise them before they come.

In having the qualities of humility and simplicity you can consider that you have everything you want; there is nothing more.

Purity weaves destiny

doubt\temptation\fear\guilt\laziness\ego

jealousy\comparison\prejudice\love\patience\tolerance

acceptance\faith\discipline\humility

Now, what are the good things that can perpetuate our purity or make it more intense? Can you identify your friends in this way? Love is number one. Patience - yes, tolerance, acceptance, faith, discipline - yes, acceptance! You have a whole list of friends.

In the *Bhagavad Gita*, Lord Krishna mentions the twenty-one or twenty-three great qualities we must have in life when we have to tackle all this warfare. I don't know why he likes to quote life as a war. He says to consider this life as being protected by a palace in which you are living, protected by a compound wall with these twenty-one or

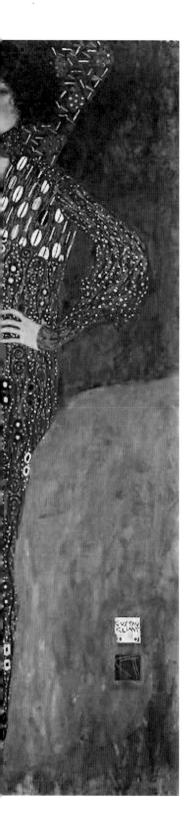

twenty-three qualities or gates. Then he says that all these gates should be protected with the lese great qualities. But it is at the back gate, which is the most vulnerable in a palace (nobody pays attention to the back gate), from which most enemies attack. From the most unexpected place they will attack. And he says that this gate must be protected always by humility. If you don't have humility, all other gates are vulnerable.

In the ten maxims, whilst ending the last maxim, the wise man mentions these particular qualities of humility and simplicity very highly. He says in having the qualities of humility and simplicity you can consider that you have everything you want; there is nothing more. In a person with humility and heart, there is not only respect, unspoken respect, but they are highly regal. The way that person conducts himself or herself, they stand out like royalty when they are walking around. You can distinctly mark that they must be of royal descent. They have that something in them.

A spiritual person also, if he has this spiritual royalty or regal quality, it will shine through when he walks or talks, or even when he does not walk or talk. There is immense courtesy and civility in the conversation. In Sahaj Marg, We not only strive for proper communication. But we go further into a state of communion from communication to communion.

Everything must be towards excellence, but without being exclusive. The exclusivity principle will destroy us. In one of the messages, it says that as long as we think ourselves to be great we continue to form the wall of greatness around us and separate ourselves from the rest of the godly kingdom. We jail ourselves. We are alone. We are alone among loved ones.

Source: From Gustav Klimt

It is only when we break the wall of greatness and submit ourselves as humble insignificant servants of the Master, of god, and only when we become nothing, subduing our tendencies and allowing him to take charge of our existence, that life will be truly enjoyable. That means total surrender.

Who wants surrender willingly? That is where the ego comes. But that is where you can also pamper your ego and say, "I will excel in my surrender." It will help and then you slowly say goodbye to it.

Naturalness

Purity does not have to be talked about. Love does not have to be talked about. It impresses your heart, unknowingly, without words. Does the rose ask whether it should radiate its fragrance? Yet, my intellect asks me, "Should I do this or should I do that?" When my inner nature is to emit purity and love all the time, where is the question of limiting myself by saying, "OKAY, I'll just be doing this at this particular time?" That wouldn't be natural. Then, I would be like those artificial perfume pumps. Have you seen those? When you pass by, they recognise your presence and emit a burst of fragrance.

Truthfulness

If I remain artificial and untruthful, I cannot even have a relationship with my wife, my family members or my friends, because I am always lying, I am always trying to impress people. There is no need to impress anyone whom are you trying to fool?

We require a lot of effort to become unnatural. To speak a lie needs a lot of effort, and you have to remember it too. To speak a lie you must be so creative, but to speak the truth you must be simple. The truth is pure, coming straight from your heart. God showers such people with so much love. They are

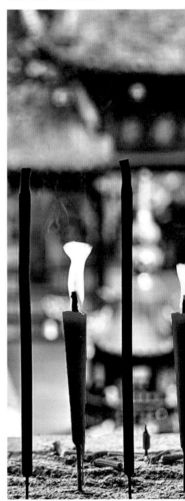

Copyright: Wang Ruiguang

content in their simplicity and purity. They are not trying to impress anyone, because they know what they are. Masters are like that, you see. They don't want to impress anybody. They are what they are.

Miseries

What is the difference between coal and a diamond? Both are carbon. When coal comes under intense pressure and heat it becomes a diamond. Our existence is like this too, yet we don't want to go through miseries, though we know very well that the end product is always good. Your childhood experiences or even your present day experiences will show you that we often talk very fondly about the miserable times. "I walked all the way to the airport." We also boast about them. There would be nothing to boast about if we had gone in a car.

When you really had a tough time and you survived with integrity, you can say, "Wow, I did It!" Tough times really do make us stronger. If you were not given any examinations in class, would you even attend classes? Perhaps very few of you, who are really sincere about education would say, "Examinations, or no examinations, I've got to study." This is a different breed of human beings. But we are afraid of tests and exams.

If we are given the opportunity, we won' t take the exam, right? That is the problem we have to correct. We need to replicate the same thing in life. Life is full of exams, full of different types of tests. Masters are also not spared from any tests. These tests are not like examinations where you are tested on your abilities. Challenges in life prepare us to do something greater.

When untoward things happen in life, we must learn from those moments. Instead of fighting, learn from them. Try to solve those problems without getting frustrated. If we get frustrated, our minds will be disturbed when he very radar, the very guide that is within us is disturbed, there will not be guidance from within. We will not be able to make the right decisions. So when challenges are there, we have to become extra alert in a very nice way. Instead of fighting, invite it.

That is why we say again and again, "Accept miseries." Not accepting them, we will never understand their purpose. What could they have done for us to where could they have taken us, to what levels? All these things will be missed out the moment we reject certain unwanted things in life. Go through it peacefully, with a quiet heart, with a bold heart, though with a lot of courage. Once you go through certain situations in life, you will emerge stronger than you were before.

If you don' t accept them, you will not learn anything. If you merely accept, you will remain a mere human being. Let's accept all these situations joyfully and cheerfully and see the beauty that emerges after that.

This requires a lot of courage and self-confidence. Then you will come out a winner. You may fail, but in the exam of life you have passed, and that's what is wanted. We don' t run away like cowards. We face life as it comes and we move on like that and that' s how we build our destiny. Unlike many others who run away from life, we face life with courage and confidence.

We all go through ordeals in life, difficulties in life, and no one is an exception to it. The difference between a normal human being and a divine purusha, is only this: that they are able to accept their difficulties and their ordeals with a smile. We cannot.

"Ordeals accept cheerfully will serve their purpose." Otherwise, for ordeals that you have to go through no matter what, whenever you accept them or not, they will not serve the purpose, and you will only suffer and no good result can come out of this process. Ordeals accepted cheerfully, going through the process, will bear spiritual fruits. So we have to accept them.

A person who goes on anticipating better moments can never be happy. You accept this and make peace with the world, make peace with yourself and that is the end of your life. You have mastered your life.

You can confidently, gracefully walk through any situation in life without being touched; Without being touched means without absorbing any impression, either on yourself or on another person. You are not creating impressions on yourself, but not on others as well. Your existence doesn't create ripples any more. If at all, it sends out waves of purity, of love, because creating impressions on others also is a problem.

Urgency

Whatever you have to do, whatever you can accomplish, finish it now while you have the strength and the stamina, especially the main thing - God Realisation. You have time to read books, you have time to acquire knowledge, you

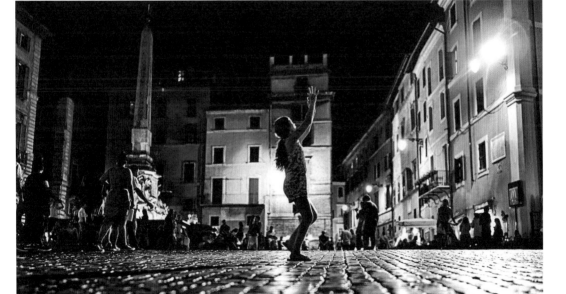

have time to sit, meditate and receive transmission, Grace and blessings from above. A time will come when you will be starving for those things, and you will say, "Oh, my pains!" Even in bed you won't have peace! How will you sit and meditate or accept transmission in that supine position? It will be very difficult, because you will be extremely engaged with your physical problems. So let's achieve what we have to achieve now, at any cost, instead of postponing it till later in life.

You must set goals for yourself. You don't have to mention them to anyone, but set your own goals and see that you achieve those goals. With each small step we take toward achieving those goals, our willpower will become stronger and stronger. Sometimes we set very high goals. Don't do such things. Take a little bit at a time - something that your mind can take, that your heart can accept. Set up smaller goals in life, but always have a focus on the main goal. All this must bring me to the highest. The highest is God Realisation, the merger.

Sleep

If people were to discipline their lives just a bit with their sleep cycles their lives could be changed. Just regularise your life, discipline your life, with these two aspects: first, sleep well, sleep by 9 o' clock.

So start with your sleep cycle. Sleep early. I may sound stupid and you may be saying, "Another preacher is here." But there are serious repercussions if you don't discipline your sleep cycle, because it is like an inner butterfly effect. You have heard that theory, no? A butterfly flaps its wings in South America, in the Amazon, and one leaf starts fluttering, two leaves start, three start and there is a snowstorm created in North America. A little discipline in how well you can sleep, how deeply you can sleep, determines your daily state of mind throughout the day.

So the choice is yours. Do you want to lead your life like

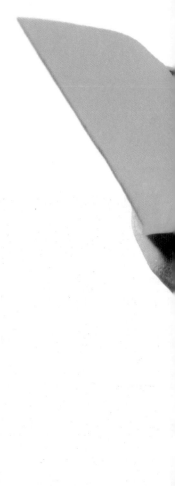

the roaring oceans, which are so pleasing to so many people today? You can never know anything that is happening there. You are lost in the waves of your disturbed consciousness. But when the consciousness is settled, even the slightest change or variation is noticed; the way even the fall of the lightest leaf can create waves. They are felt. On the other hand, the poor rock in the ocean - nothing happens to it. That is why friends get along, because they are like oceans. They fight with each other and nothing happens. But in a love relationship, if you even look at a person like this, it creates a wave, "Oh! He looked at me like this today." It is something to think about.

There is a beautiful statement in our first maxim where it says that you can swim with the river's flow. You can also swim against the flow, but it will consume you.

In our yogic shastras, great significance was given to both nostrils. In the yogic shastras, the right nostril is considered to be Surya Nadi. It is called Pingala. The left nostril is considered to be Ida and it is dominant during the night. It is called Chandra Nadi. Ideally, the right nostril should be predominant during the daytime and the left nostril should be predominant at night. Why? Well, we don't have much time for all those whys and hows, but let's just remember this: the impact on our physiology is directly related to the movement of both the sun and moon. When something is not right, a switch occurs.

So that is why in the olden days they would get up and examine their breathing. If their breathing was not as it should be, then they would drink some hot water and do things like pranayama, walking, etc. if you are very careful, just around sunrise and sunset you will witness a slow shift from right to left, or left to right. And if you happen to meditate at that time, I tell you that it will be like a rocket as it is just the right time, because the balance there between your sympathetic and parasympathetic system.

Now what happens to people who go to bed very late at night? Watch this, when you go to sleep on time, by 9 o'clock or 10 o'clock, and observe the right nostril switch to the left and the left to the right. If you get the right amount of sleep, your right nostril will automatically be predominant in the morning as soon as you get up. Over millennia, actually, our systems have evolved in such a way that when the sun rises certain hormonal patterns are triggered. If you follow the rhythm, then your health will automatically improve. If you go against the rhythm, it is like swimming against the current, which will consume you over time. When your strength and youthfulness start to decline, then you will be swimming against the current and your decline in health will speak volumes. It is better to set a pattern now.

I think nightly activities are a curse of the modern world. Because of electricity, there isn't now much difference between day and night. Starved sleep patterns reflect irregularities and your health suffers because of that. Your immunity levels also go down because the nervous system is breaking down.

Extensive studies have been conducted on people who work at night, especially those who do not have any choice, who would otherwise remain jobless. If you observe their health patterns, you will find their ageing to be very rapid. Most of us are not working at night. We have a choice, yet our lifestyle is like those who are helpless, who must work at night. We volunteer to stay awake all night, watching all kinds of stuff.

So either way you look at it, whether spiritually or health-wise, it is a self - defeating purpose. So why indulge? What is the point of doing such business where there is only loss. So go to sleep early, please. It will help us a lot.

In Gujarati, we have a saying: "one who goes to bed early and wakes up early increases their physical strength, mental intellect and remains prosperous." These are words of wisdom.

Only a healthy body can have a healthy mind and vice versa. A lot of people make the argument that a healthy mind makes for a healthy body, but without also having a healthy body, your mind will go crazy. "Oh, my legs are not working, my hands are not working and so many other things are not working." You go to doctors, you start worrying and you go crazy. How are you going to build your destiny? You have already chosen a destructive path, simply by not following the natural rhythm.

One of our maxims says to be in tune with nature. You will get nothing by resisting. There is a beautiful statement in our first maxim where it says that you can swim with the rivers flow. You can also swim against the flow, but it will consume you. Early in the morning, nature's energy flows in one direction towards the source. It is not a physical energy. It is best when you are flowing with those currents. But as I told you

Source: From the Internet

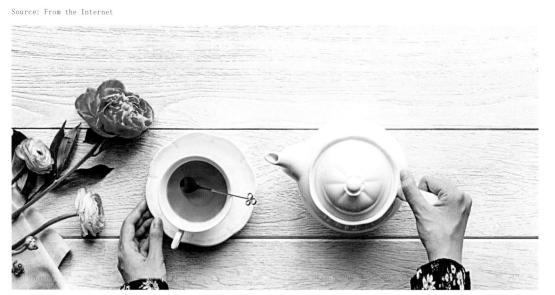

177

yesterday, one dose and you are knocked out because of your weakness.

So if you want to go further, you must adjust your sleep patterns at any cost. Otherwise, you will struggle with that one fundamental thing all your life. You will wake up frustrated and sleepless. You won't be able to meditate properly. If you cannot meditate properly, you won't have a proper spiritual condition to work with. You won't have a proper consciousness to begin with, even for mundane things. You have uprooted your consciousness, the very guiding force. You have exposed yourself to so many things. You are now vulnerable. More and more, you become a garbage collector, collecting impressions throughout the day, and it is a whole vicious cycle.

Per contra, if you have a fine condition, a pure condition, a blissful condition, you are more grateful. This gratitude emerging from the heart creates a bond between our maker and you. There is great benefit in this, and as you get more and more benefit, you feel like doing more and more.

认识旅程
Understanding the Journey

跟随心

印度有一首歌里这样唱道:

"人们为何走走停停才能稳定脚步,

既然提心吊胆,何苦出家门,

为何每次转弯都瞻前顾后脚步才能稳定。"

相信这也是歌者在用他的方式表达跟随心的重要性。

上天给了我们一颗心,不论事情好坏,这颗心都会做出回应。出现不好的事情它就会发出信号:"这样不对。"至于这个信号到底发自心还是发自头脑,请不要想太多。如果正确地经过思维过程,也会引导我们达到与心相同的结论,但关键是有没有迈出正确的、符合逻辑的步骤。让我们不要分开心脑,就把它们当作事物的两面,并倾听这个声音,而不被错误的行为带走。

心和头脑会告诉我们有哪一点不好、不自然。至于好的、自然的东西从来不会有任何信号。我们可以观察一些生活中最平常的例子,来验证这一情况。当呼吸正常时,没有问题。我也不会有疑问。我的心不会跟我说:"好棒!你的呼吸正常呢!"而一旦呼吸失常、视力减弱或有任何不自然的事情发生时,心马上就会给出信号。撒谎时，心马上就会有信号，而说真话则属于自然，心不会吭声。

再比如，关于伴侣的选择问题，一旦你的心中提问，"对我而言，这个人是对的吗？"这些问题多半本身就是一种信号。有对的人在你面前，你不会有任何疑问。心中不会出现哪怕一丝的怀疑，你会勇往直前。但请不要开始分析："他的月薪多少？""他的母亲会怎么待我？"这样你就坏事了。有一首歌说的是："不要探试人家，试探的就不再是自己人。"

为何我们常常无法做到跟随心？

我们的探讨会从两个故事开始：

故事一

你在花园中散步，一朵玫瑰花的芬芳让你印象深刻，然后你继续向前走。第二天当你经过那里的时候你就敏感于那种宜人的芬芳，主动去寻找。你说"哇，真美"，然后继续往前走。第三天，也许会走过去观赏或捧在手中，"实在太美了"。第四天你可能干脆把它摘下来带回家。

故事二

有一个圣人在森林里宁静地冥想。他没有任何烦恼，时刻处于喜悦之中，也备受邻近村民的尊重。他只有一块腰布，每晚他就把腰布洗好，晾在树枝上。但有一些老鼠开始咬这块腰布，因此腰布变得越来越小。村民们这就提议"给您买只猫吧"，他们买了只猫给他，以便赶走老鼠。但是养猫还要不停地喂牛奶，因此有人开始每晚带牛奶

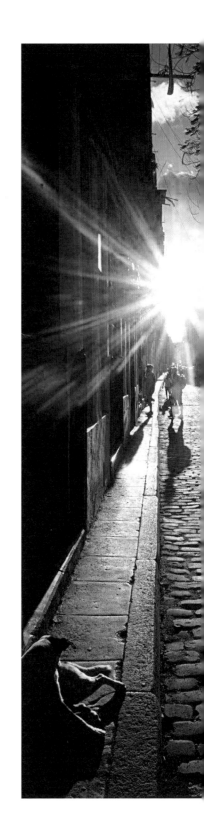

过来喂猫，直到厌倦了他们就说："怎么能每晚冒着生命危险过来，还要赶回去？"因此，他们决定买头牛给他。这下需要有人懂得挤奶来喂猫以便抓老鼠，他们就派了个女佣去挤奶。最后圣人爱上了女佣，就与她成家了。

　　不知在阅读完你们是否有些发现呢？两个故事有着惊人的相似，都是从一件小事开始，引发了如此大的连锁反应：在故事一中，我们一次闻到芬芳还不满足，发出了"美妙，上天好伟大"的赞叹后，还想拥有，想要占有；在故事二中，圣人一直很满足，但有一个小小的欲望就打破了一切。当我们偏离以爱生活的原则时，当我们偏离简单、朴素的原则时，就会走上不自然的生活。不自然的生活即不断制造心灵印记。我们可以观察日常生活最让我们印象深刻的事情，并尝试去探索是一些什么样的印记主宰着我们的生活以及这些印记形成背后的机制究竟为何：是一些什么样的行动、不行动、思想以及行为产生印记？有时候我们甚至可能没有参与其中，但依然产生了印记，比如有件事情本应该做，应该在某某时候做好，我们却没有做。这种事情会让我们毕生不得安宁。

　　当今时代的大环境，也在我们偏离纯净内心的路上助了一臂之力！其中一大祸害是电视和电脑，它们扮演什么角色呢？就是不断提醒我们自己缺少什么："哦，你没有这个"，提醒你"你的老公可没有这种表示"或"你的丈夫是这样的"或"你的老婆是这样的"。提醒你："你没有这样的房子，没有这种电视机，没有这样的知心朋友，没尝过这种美酒佳肴，没有去过某某地方旅游。"但我们的真心并不提醒我们缺点什么，是她让我们变得没有缺乏，变得轻而易举地富足，前提是我们能够跟随心。

如何能做到跟随心？

（一）转向自己

认清假设很重要。我们日夜见人，想象着各种情况，并不停地积累心灵印记。但是在积累心灵印记之前，我们在内心不断做出假设："看他的衬衣，哪儿买的？""啊，她的衣服可没那么好。""讲师心情好像没那么好。""我今天心情很差。"虽然没有说出口，但我们一直不停地在假设。

那么这种不断地假设各样事情，尤其是负面的事情，有什么帮助呢？比如说，我们无法想象恒河第一次从恒河源头渗出来的

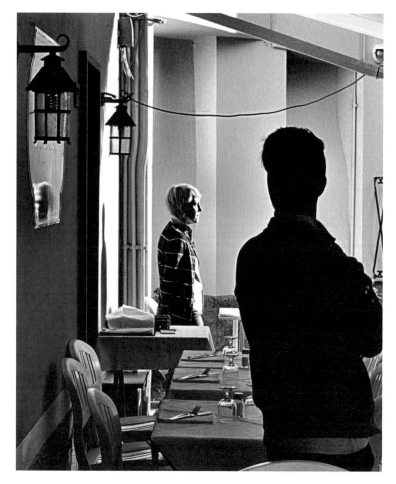

照片：王锐光摄

样子，但是假如有能力跟随第一滴水而行，会很奇妙——发现它遇到了什么样的阻力，然后如何绕道而行，最终流入大洋。假如能步步跟随，该多么美妙。

同样，我们可以看着自己的意念在自己的心中诞生，然后看看其去向，尤其是我们的状态。正如那条河流那样，意念会化为较强的东西并加强状态。当不能再用言语解释时，我们就沉浸于内心的最新状态，毕竟我们就是要学习心的语言。但是假如你说："这里这样，那里那样，他有这款手表，她有苹果手机"，那就完了。你的注意力始终被外在的事物所吸引，处于这样的状态时，我们就没有办法把一点点的注意力给到内心，更何况倾听心的声音。

（二）态度

任何一项练习都是一种劳作过程，能将爱、谦卑与祈祷带进来就会有帮助。你在戏院外等女朋友，她却迟迟不到，在开场前五分钟才到达，此时你会如何呢？简直好像经过了永久的时间："你怎么现在才到！"你会变得如此忐忑不安。接下来我们会分享另一些故事来说明为什么需要对练习培养这种着迷、激情以及忐忑的态度。否则，练习没有用。只是劳作，枯燥之味，也因此而没有收获。

你们可见过农场的工人？他在挣每日的工钱。而比如有人去健身房，可能每天只花半个小时的时间却能练出肌肉。农场的工人整天都在劳作，但不停地诅咒自己"我得干活，我得干活"，然后肌肉全没了。还是态度的问题。如果觉得练习枯燥乏味，然后不停地诅咒："哦，我又要做这个，爸爸，妈妈。"如果只是为了满足家人，不如不做。不适合你还是放弃好了。否则你闭着眼睛浪费那么多时间，也没有什么收获，也赚不到什么东西，有何意义？当你做一件事的时候，应当愉悦地去做。

进化

我们在中、小学和大学都学过进化的过程；达尔文理论以及适应和突变理论。但那些讲的都是形态的变化、细胞的变化。当然，这些也都很重要。最近有一些研究表明，环境对基因的变异也有自身的影响。我可以举一个简单的例子，这个例子来自我读过的一本叫做《信仰生理学》的书，作者是布鲁斯·利普顿博士。他举了在破碎家庭中长大的孩子或婴儿的例子，家里总是有人争吵，十分不和谐。就像在纽约布鲁克林，有些社区整晚都是枪声不绝于耳。准妈妈们时刻处于压力之下。如果去审视面对暴力威胁的生理反应，我们会发现什么呢？假如有人要攻击你，你会怎么办？如果有能力也许会和他对打，不然就逃离现场避免打架。不论如何，逃跑也需要力量。所以作者说要么打，要么逃之夭夭，两种情况都需要肢体。因此，血液会更多地在肢体中循环，远离了如胃、肾、脾、肺和大脑等内脏器官。

当妈妈们时刻处于压力之下时会怎么样？液总是往肢体流。血液中收缩剂和刺激质得到刺激，而体内的胚胎也会有相同的反应，胎儿肢体中的血液会比内脏多。因此这种孩子生下来之后四肢会比一般人长。这里发生的第二件事是大脑后叶和前叶在发育中出现差异。前叶负责认知。有机会在健康家庭、有爱的环境下成长时，胎儿

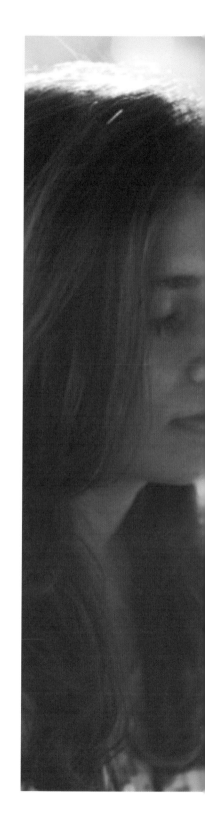

会培养各种直觉本能。当没有爱和关心时，后叶会变得较大，因为血液一直往那边流。但是我们会说：父亲大脑发育良好，肢体正常，妈妈肢体也正常，大脑的大小良好，那么胎儿为什么没有相同的基因模式出现？肢体变得比较长，消化系统发育欠佳。由此可见，基因上胎儿得到了正确的编码，但环境改变了编码并让内脏器官以这种方式成长。因此，环境对基因的形式有一定的，甚至可以说永久且不可逆转的作用。

那么当我们冥想的时候，实际上在发生什么呢？有人已经做过一些试验，参与试验的有冥想了约五万个小时的人。纵观一个人的寿命，其实这还不算多。试验结果表明，这些人当中大脑髓鞘比较厚。多了兆亿胞突结合和神经元；即便只增加一毫米的厚度，也会有数十亿个额外胞突结合。另外发现，有规律冥想的人大脑前叶高度发达；这里说的有规律不是指每天五分钟。较长的时间以及频率较高，则效果不样。因此冥想本身对我们的生理系统有一定的影响。即便不是心灵成长上，但在情绪上以及生理上我们也会变得更好一些。

振动兼容性

兼容是一个极度精妙的概念。当你在服用某种药物时，假如偶然服用了一些与那个药物不兼容的东西，身体内部就会发生冲突。似乎发生了大战，而我们会因此而痛苦。

兼容也是人际中系中的一个因素。对人类而言，问题是如何与所有人培养兼容性？经过三十午的相处，我与我

照片来源于《满心》杂志

185

妻子的关系可以调整好。同样，随着孩子的成长，其行为模式也会开始得到表现，我们开始习惯于彼此，或许需要25年吧。商业伙伴，工作同事或学校里面都有各种振动层次。你可以与这个层次或那个层次互动，但本身都不兼容。如何让所有这些振动层次与自己的振动层次相匹配呢？

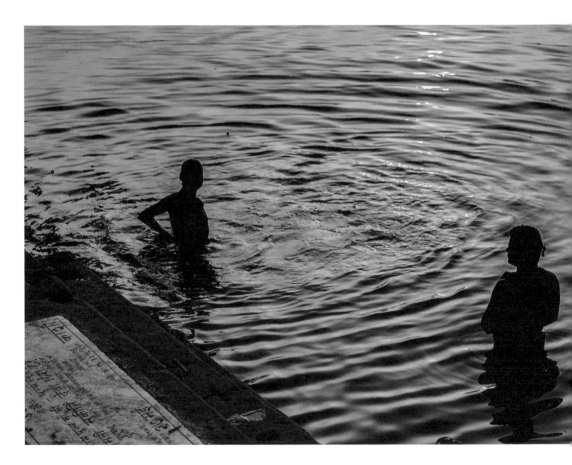

Following the heart

There are lyrics from a famous Indian song.

Why do people tread so cautiously?

If they are so afraid, why do they step out of their homes in the first place?

Why do people hesitate at every turn?

God has given us a heart that responds to everything, good and bad. The moment anything wrong happens, it gives us a signal: "this is not right." Don't think too much about whether the signal is coming from the heart or the mind. If you follow the intellectual process properly, it will also lead you to the same result as the heart, but the key is whether you have taken the right steps, the logical steps. Let's not differentiate between the heart and mind. Let's see this as a spectrum of consciousness with two ends. Listen to it and don't get carried away by the wrong activity.

The heart and mind always signal us as to what is wrong, what is unnatural. They will never give us the signal for what is right, because what is right is natural. You may not understand this, but let me give you an example in our daily life. When I am breathing properly, nothing is wrong. I don't question myself. My heart is not telling me, "You are breathing well. Well done!" But the moment my breathing suffers, the moment my eyesight suffers, the moment anything unnatural happens, the heart will give us an immediate signal. When we speak a lie, it gives an immediate signal. When we speak the truth it is natural. The heart doesn't have to say anything.

Any time you question, "this person right or wrong for me?" most of the time the questions themselves are a signal. When the right person comes before

照片来源于网络

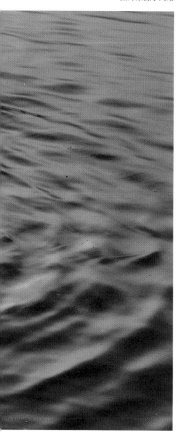

you, you will have no doubt. Not even a single doubt will arise in your heart. You will just go ahead. But then, don't start analysing, "How much will his salary be? How will his mother be?" Then you are spoiling it. There is a ghazal that goes, "Don't put someone to the test. When you do that, they are no longer yours."

Why can't we follow the heart?

We start our discussion with 2 stories.

Story 1:

Perhaps you are walking in a garden and are impressed by the nice fragrance of a rose, and then you continue on your way. The next day when you walk past, you become alert to the beautiful fragrance there. You look for it. "Ah, it's beautiful", you say, and then you walk on. On the third day, you want to go nearer and hold it. "Oh, it's so beautiful." On the fourth day, you pluck it and take it home. This is how we form impressions. We are not happy with one inhalation and, "It's wonderful, God is great!" We want to own it. We want to possess it. Then the problem starts.

Story 2:

There was a beautiful story about a saint who was peacefully meditating in a jungle. He had no problems. He was blissful and well respected by the villagers nearby. He had only one loincloth to worry about, which he would wash and hang on a tree branch at night. But these little mice started eating it while it hung on the branch and his loincloth was slowly becoming smaller and smaller. So the villagers suggested, "Let's get you a cat." They got him a cat to chase away the mice, but to keep a cat you have to give it milk all the time. So somebody started bringing milk every evening to feed the cat until they got tired of it. They said, "How can we come every evening and

Source: From the Internet

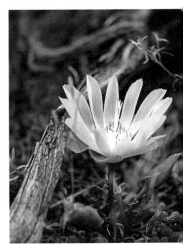

risk our lives returning back to the village?" So they decided to get him a cow. Now somebody needed to milk the cow, to feed the cat, to run after the mice. They sent a maid to milk the cow. He fell in love with that maid and started a family.

What a small thing triggered such a chain reaction! The nice fragrance is not enough. The desire of owning and possessing it starts the problem. The saint had been perfectly happy, but one little desire and there it went. When we deviate from this principle of leading a life with love, we tend to lead an unnatural life. An unnatural life means the formation of samskaras, the formation of impressions. In my day-to-day observations of life, what is it that strikes me the most? What sort of samskaras dominate in our lives, and what is the mechanism by which these samskaras are formed? What sort of actions, inactions, thoughts and behaviours? Many a time we may not even be a part of it, and yet we may end up forming samskaras. Such things haunt us all our lives.

The modern disease of the TV and computer, what do they do actually? They remind us of our incompleteness: "Oh, you don't have this." It reminds you that, "Your husband is not behaving like this." or "Your husband is like this." or "your wife is like this." It reminds you that, "you don't have a house like this, you don't have a TV like this, you don't have friends like this, you don't have food like this, you haven't visited such-and-such a tourist place." But our heart doesn't remind us of our incompleteness; it completes us, provided we obey.

How can we follow the heart?

1. Reorienting towards the self

It is very important to understand suppositions. Day and night we meet people and we imagine things, gathering impressions all the time. But prior to gathering these impressions, we continuously go on supposing things within ourselves. "Look at his shirt-where did he buy it from?" "Oh, her cloth is not so good." "The lecturer is not in good spirits." "My mood is not good today." We are all continuously supposing things inside even without being vocal. We are busy in the wrong things.

So this continuous supposing of things, especially negative things, how does it help us? For example, we cannot imagine what it would have been like to have seen the river Ganga for the first time coming from its source, when it was first created and trickling down. But if we had had the opportunity of walking along with the first drop, it would have been wonderful — the kind of resistance it encountered and then how it went around, ultimately meeting the ocean. If we could have followed it, it would have been wonderful.

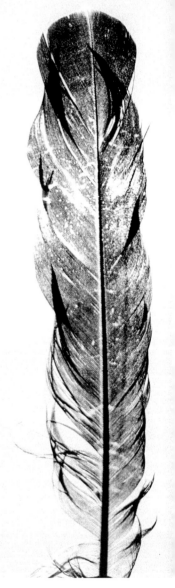

Likewise, we can watch the moment our ideas take birth in our heart and see where they go, especially our condition. Like a river flowing, ideas evolve into something greater and reinforce the condition. When nothing further is explainable by words, you are lost into your own Self with a newer condition, because you are occupied with your inner studies. But if you are, "Oh, here this is happening, that is happening, he has this watch, he has that iPhone," all labour is lost in that. Your attention is occupied with external things. In such condition, we can't pay attention to our heart or listen to the heart.

2. Attitudes

Any practice in itself is a labour process. Bringing in the attitudes of love, humility and prayerfulness helps. When you wait for your girlfriend by the theatre and she doesn't show up and she comes just five minutes before the movie begins, what happens? It feels like eternity: "You didn't come on time!" You become so restless. I will share some other anecdotes, some stories, and explain to you why we must create fascination, passion and restlessness toward the practice itself. Otherwise there is no point practicing – it is a labour, it is a dry practice, and you don't earn anything.

Have you seen a labourer on the farm? He is earning his daily wages. But a man who goes to the gym, for example, may be spending just over half an hour a day and he builds up muscles. The man on the farm works the whole day, but he is cursing himself, "I have to work, I have to work," and he loses his muscles. It is a matter of attitude again. If you think your practice is a dry thing, and you curse, "Oh, I have to do it again, papa, mama." If you are doing it just to satisfy some of your family members, it is better that you don't do it. It is not for you, so drop it. Otherwise you are wasting so much time with your eyes closed, not getting anything, not earning anything. What is the point? When you do something, you must do it joyfully and cheerfully.

Evolution

We have been taught in schools and colleges about the evolutionary path; Darwin's theory and theories of adaptation and mutation. But that is all about morphological change, cellular change. That too is very important. There are recent discoveries where the environment has its own effect on genetic manipulation. I'll give you a small example from a book I read *The Biology of Belief* by Dr Bruce Lipton. He gives the example of a child or a baby that is conceived in a broken family where there is always a fight in the house, and there is total discord. It is like Brooklyn, where gunshots are heard all around at night in some places. The mother-to-be is always under stress. Now what happens if you look at the physiological response to violence? If somebody tries to attack me, what do I do? If I have strength, I'll fight back or I'll run away from the scene so I don't have to fight. Nevertheless even to run I need strength. So he says that either you fight or you take flight. Under both circumstances you need your limbs. So blood circulates more into the limbs and away from the visceral organs like the stomach, liver, spleen, lungs and brain.

What happens when mothers are always under stress? The blood flow is always towards the limbs. The agonists, the stimulators are triggered into the blood, and the foetus that is growing within as an embryo also responds accordingly. The blood in the foetus' limbs will be greater than the visceral organs. So the limbs of such children when they are born are longer than other normal human beings.

The second thing that happens is there is a difference in the growth of the posterior lobe and the frontal lobe of the brain. The frontal lobe is for cognition. Intuitive faculties develop when the foetus gets a chance to grow healthy family environment where there is love and affection. Where there is none, the back part grows much bigger because all the time the blood flow is only going there.

But we say: the father's brain is well developed his limbs are normal, and the mothers limbs are normal, and the size of her brain is well developed, so how come the same genetic pattern did not allow the foetus to grow accordingly, but differently? The limbs are longer and the digestive system is suffering because the digestive organs did not develop so well. So genetically the foetus actually received the proper code, but it is the environment that changed the code and permitted the organs to develop the way they did. So the environment has a definite effect, a permanent irreversible effect on genetic patterns.

When we meditate, what really happens? They have done experiments on people who have meditated for let us say 50,000 hours. It is not much actually when you see the lifespan of a person. The layer that they call the myelin sheath is thicker. There are trillions of synapses and billions of neurons; even if it grows by one millimetre thickness it will still have billions of extra synapses. Also, the frontal lobes are very well developed in people who are meditating regularly; not just regularly for five minutes every day. Longer periods with frequent meditations also have a different sort of effect. So meditation itself has a definite effect on our physiological system. If not spiritually, at least emotionally, and physically also we will be better.

Vibratory compatibility

Compatibility is an extremely superfine concept. When you are taking one medication, if by accident you take something that is not compatible with that drug there is a clash inside. There is a world war and you suffer as a result of it.

Compatibility is also an issue in human relationships. For human beings, the question is how to develop compatibility with one and all at the same time? I can become adjusted with my wife over a period of thirty years of association. Similarly, as children grow up, their behavior manifests. We get used to each other. It takes perhaps twenty-five years. With business partners in the work environment, or in a school or college, wherever you are, there is an entire gamut of vibratory levels. You can try to interact with this level and with that level, and everything is incompatible perse. How do I make all vibratory levels match with my own?

Source: From the Internet

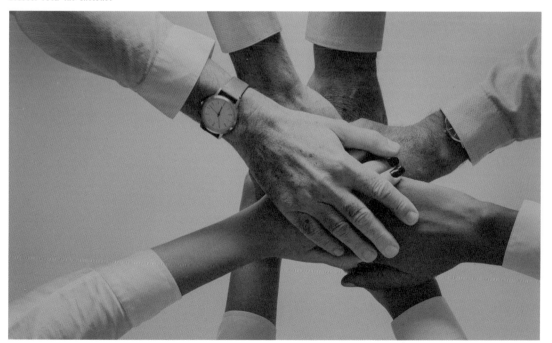

人际关系
Relationships

尊重他人

如有国王接见，你会不会穿短裤前往？不会。为什么呢？因为你要表达对国王的尊重。这背后的原则并不是想打扮得漂亮一点。我每天都想好看一点，但访问有一定地位的人时需要格外小心。我打领带去上班，是因为有客户来访，并不是想炫耀自己的领带。穿着得体恰恰就是为了表达对他人的尊重。不是为自己，而是为他人。

我说话礼貌，即便没有说话，只是默默地坐在房间里，我的坐姿、举止也都会向他人表达一点什么。有客人在面前而我却弯腰垂头，这样并不礼貌。尽管没有说出一句话，但你也是不尊重大家。你说，"你今天很好看，亲爱的"，但话没说完人就走了。你到底为什么要开口？或者用很飘忽的神情看着别人，以这样的方式表达自己。你的表情也能表达一点什么。

有些人走进一个房间的时候好像带来了风暴，门"砰"的一声关闭。也许一句话没说，但走路的样子、说话的声音、一举一动都能反映很多问题。他们带着一种目中无人的气势，因为对他人没有爱，没有尊重。尊重实际上是内心有爱的表现。你不爱自己，这种情操就永远养不成。换一个角度去看，你生气是因为发生了事情，让你心中不喜欢。此时，你能尊重他人吗？恐怕不能。

但处于爱的状态时，即便是你敌人来到面前，由于你的样子，他会觉得"太好了!我们还是朋友"。离开时人已经不一样了。

我们每一天都在与那么多人互动，老的少的都有。跟小孩子互动时，我们有时候不够小心，会去戏弄他们，觉得只是孩子嘛。但我观察过智者们，即便与小孩交流时都会用"您"来称呼对方。甚至幼辈他都如此地尊重。当你如此尊重一个小孩时，也会在他心中唤起这种品质，帮助他学会为人处世。但设若不停地重复，"笨蛋，坐下，你不应该这样，应该那样"，不停地责骂、嘲弄，把人逼到角落，那么他也会学会以相同的方式说话。毕竟从很小的时候，对他而言，尊重的概念就变得很陌生。

小孩不懂什么叫尊重是因为大人不尊重小孩。即便他们只是有个小小想法，觉得"哇，这朵花好漂亮"，就应该赞扬他，说："瞧!真的好漂亮，你说得对。"引导孩子进一步去探索。"你看看有多少花瓣?是什么颜色的?香不香?"培养其分析能力。从零开始，然后看看能把我们带到哪儿去。

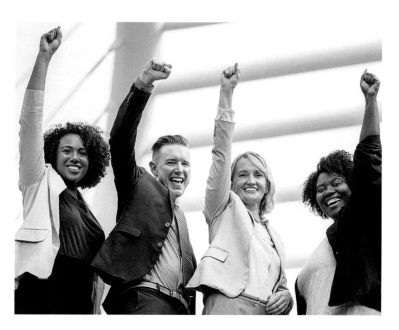

照片来源于网络

人际关系中的熵

何谓熵?

让我们用比较实际的方式去理解这个概念。比如说你从图书馆借了一本书回来,然后你的父亲又赠送一本书给你作为礼物。你的女朋友给了你一些杂志,你自己也有一些音乐碟片。所有这些东西都堆在你房间的一个小桌子上。房间别的地方也一片狼藉,衣服在这里,袜子在那里,毛巾又挂在某处。这是个分解的系统;系统已经陷入混乱之中。

这种混乱不堪让你受不了,你就开始收拾房间:每一本书放到正确的位置,衣服洗好,床也收拾好。这下房间看起来比以前干净了,直到你又开始把书或别的东西带回来,系统又开始重新分解并走向混沌。要维持秩序的话,就需要能量不断输入。

因此,熵指的是任何系统中混乱的程度。热力学第二定律认为熵随时间而增加。这反映的是假如没有稳定因素,随着时间的推移,系统将出现不稳定。

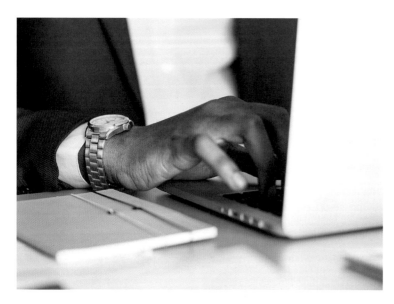

照片来源于网络

在人际关系中，我们日复一日地互动，这些关系也就逐渐变得乱七八糟。我们任由一些东西在内室中堆积，这些内室随着堆积程度而变得越来越混乱，正如房间里的书籍和衣物一样。我们总是耿耿于怀，除非采取措施，否则有朝日必然导致爆炸。任何关系想要稳定的话，就需要有输入来熨平皱褶或分歧，以便不再无休止地积累东西。

难道每次犯错误都需要这样吗？是不是每次都要拿冰激凌或甜食来安慰人？这就意味着在不断付出来维持一种关系。

假如每逢与亲友争吵或争论都需要不断输入，那么每次将会需要比上次更多的输入。甚至假如能够买得起的话，有天可能要买辆奔驰给他们！同时，不论需要付出什么代价，我们都应该相爱。在这个过程中无疑会受伤，也会消耗很多力量；但如果准备好去面对，你的关系就会得到改善。

在家庭中，如果需要彼此容忍，那就需要不断输入。需要不断输入感情的地方，即便还是在一起，也已经属于破碎的家庭。

相比之下，当成员之间有爱、有接受时，就不再需要不停地用冰激凌或是到什么世外桃源度假来维持关系。大家都用爱彼此接受，并深信对方也一样。结论是，正是心中的爱起到稳定关系的那个输入的作用。一切安好，更有较高程度的接受。

我在此谈的不是包容。包容或许是个美德，但当你觉得"我受不了这个人犯的错误"时，只有爱能熨平一切；因此，一切变得安然无事。那么这种爱究竟来自哪里？来自纯洁的心，来自真诚的心。

不信任会毒害人际关系，但是在让我们学会爱，学会牺牲，学会接受并保持这个纯洁的家庭中，我们就能放下一切。如能懂得熵的原理，就能排除不兼容。

当我的状态始终是爱时，那么不断输入就不再有必要，不断输入就会化为零输入。当只需要零输入的时候，就说明这种关系是最为稳定的关系，或者说是最为稳定的家庭。在这种家庭中不需要解释；不需要"我这么做就是因为……""我不想怎么样是因为……"有爱的地方，不需要解释。

婚姻

有些人的婚姻为什么会失败呢？我想是时候跟你们讲讲这个问题了。我们那个年代并没有人指导我们，一切都是偶然。如果去问任何人，为什么恋爱后的婚姻会失败，他们也会觉得难以解释，或者会给出各种理由。

如果两个人真正相爱，所发生的事情其实是这样的：爱出现之后，两个人的心会开始扩展，以至于能容纳对方的切。甚至连对方的错误都变得那么可爱。她啐一口痰在你身上，也没有问题。你只会洗一洗自己的衬衣或说："没事，买件新的"，不会吵架的。

然后就是第二个阶段。当你真正开始相爱时，你就会开始失去自己，开始一种自我毁灭。不论要付出什么代价，你都想让对方高兴。

但假如对方没有回报那么多，会发生什么呢？这下相爱程度开始不同，你也会开始评判："哦，可能我不应该这么做。"你开始退缩，因为你不想完全失去自己。你开始害怕。这种恐惧来自于自我。至此，你已经回忆起自己，两个人的关系就开始陷入混乱。

至此你已经开始意识到自己的需要，而之前的你完全没有这个意识。你本来想为对方付出一切。如今，你却开始想起，

"哦,我在失去自己的认识。我本来是某某身份,我可是音乐家,我可是一名医生,而如今却需要牺牲那么多。"这就是为什么两个人的关系会破裂。一旦有"我牺牲了"的念头,你的爱情故事就画上了句号。

问:那么这个问题有没有解决方案呢?择偶标准中最重要的是什么呢?

答:这个问题很难回答。或者说答案难以接受,要想付诸行动就更难了。你必须用心去想。凭我自己对人生的那么一点理解,我的答案是不要"期望过高"。这是真话。自然之道自始至终都是谈接受。而当我们学会了随遇而安的艺术,不论是面对境况、工作、生意职业还是配偶的问题,正是接受带来成功。连细菌都可以发生突变以便适应不良环境,我们为什么会做不到呢?我们需要不断适应情况,而不被其所左右。没有完美的人存在,假如那个人真的完美,还需要留在这里干什么?我们在以彼此的不完美相互碰撞。如果追求完美,首先要向自己提问:我是否完美?

社会转化

问:作为灵性寻求者,我们是否也应对国家的建设、社会的进步做一些贡献,还是只专注于个人的发展?

答:假如你想改变首都整体的人口(假如你有这个能力),但你却没有变化,请问有什么用呢?"让我去照顾下人家的妻子",可你自己的夫人却在家里受苦。因此,慷慨要从自家起步从自身起步。首先建设好自己,才能去帮助别人。你首先要有一百万美元才能给别人十万美元吧。你一无所有却有志捐赠一百万美元,纯属浮夸。说不定要抢人家的钱去给予别人。你自己得不到安宁,怎么能把这种状态反射于别人?

有些人一进教室就开始闹事。有一些教授也是这样。你心里可能想着希望这个人永远不要回来，正是因为他们所带来的气氛。这便是他们的样子。而有些老师，你很期待能与他们在一起。有些朋友，你之所以喜欢，是因为他们的那个品质。

我们在走向完美。哪方面的完美呢？不是外貌或其他迷人的东西，而是内在平衡，人格的完美，行为的无瑕。

首先我要变得完美，于内在变成一个完美的人。如果在人生每个阶段我都在期望越来越多，然后不断失望，那么也许我有些高估了自己。失望多半来自想成为与众不同。独一无二会带来很多问题："我想以独特的方式为国家服务。"谁来任命呢？先成为完美的人再说吧。

我向大家推荐印度一位智者写的关于如何迎来世界和平的信。1957年他写了这封信给联合国，并指出不仅仅是提升一个国家，而是提升全世界乃至全宇宙的方法。我们的平衡状态、内在状态，随着我们的进步会远远超于我们所在的空间，其影响范围

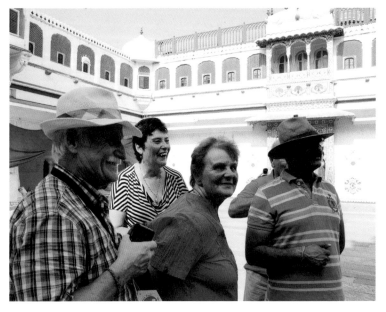

照片：那泽民摄

可以用星际来计算。

你们当中大部分人会觉得我下面要说的话与我们的问题无关，但也不是完全没有关系。测量光速的方程式是什么呢? 如果距离在零时间内穿越，这种速度叫什么? 叫无限速。那么，加入爱因斯坦的公式把能量定义为质量乘以光速的平方，如果把无限加进来，那个能量会怎么样? 我们都体验过你一想，慧能就在那里。所出现的能量是无限的，因此其能量源必须是无限的。请十分认真地思考这个问题。我完全可以用科学的方式去证明自然之道的功效。

我们至少不应让世界进一步恶化。我们尝试让环境变得清晰一些。当我们进行清心的时候，不仅在清理自己，也在为家庭的和谐做出贡献。

Respect for Others

If you visited a king, would you wear shorts? You wouldn't. Why? Because you would want to show respect to the king. The principle here is not that you want to look good. I want to look good every day but I have to be extra careful when I visit someone of a certain stature. When I wear a tie and go to the office because some guests are visiting me, I do it as a mark of respect for the others. It is not that I want to wear a tie to show off. It is precisely to show respect toward others that I dress properly. It is not for myself, it is for others.

When I speak respectfully or even if I say nothing when I am quiet in a room, the way I sit, the way I hold my head up conveys something to the people I am meeting. When a few guests are present and I am slouching, it is not respectful.

You are disrespecting everyone there - though you speak not a word, your behaviour says it. You can say, "you look good today, honey", but then you just walk off. Why did you even speak? Or you look in a very pathetic way, expressing yourself like that your looks convey something.

Some people walk into a room as if they have created a storm. They bang the doors. They may not have even spoken a word, yet the way they walk, or the way they talk, or the way they look around speaks volumes. They carry an atmosphere of disrespect, because they don't have love for others. They don't have respect for others. Respect is actually the epitome of love within oneself. If you don't love yourself, this very fine quality can never develop inside you. Look at another scenario, when you are angry. You are angry because something happened that you dislike within yourself. Can you respect others at that time? It is not possible. But when you are in a state of love, even when your enemy comes in front of you, because of the way you look he feels, "Oh good! We are still friends." He goes back changed.

We interact with so many people every single day, from children to the elderly with children many times we take it for granted, and we fool around with them, we joke around with them, thinking they are only children. But I noticed the sage's interaction even with little children, he would say "Thou". There was so much respect even for the young ones. When you address a child with a lot of respect, you are invoking that quality in that little fellow who is trying to come up in this world and grow. But if you keep on telling him, "you stupid fellow, sit down, you should not be doing this, you should not be doing that", all the time lecturing and joking and putting him in a corner, then he will learn to talk in the same way. Thus, from a very early age this idea of respect becomes foreign to him.

Children don't know what respect is because elders don't respect the younger ones. Even when they have an idea like, "Oh this flower is beautiful", at that time praise that child by saying, "Oh look! It is such a wonderful flower you are so right." Guide him further to do more research. "How many petals are there? What is the colour? How do you like the fragrance of it? " Create his analytical abilities. You start from scratch and you see where it all can go.

Entropy in Human Relationships

What is entropy?

Let's try to understand it practically you bring a book home from the library, and then your father gives you another book as a gift. Your girlfriend gives you magazines, and you have music CDs. They all pile up on a small table in your room, so now there will be enough clutter on your table. The rest of your room is also in a disorganized state, your clothes are here, your socks are there and your towel is hanging somewhere. This is a disintegrated system; the system has gone haywire.

You get frustrated with the mess and clean everything up. You put each book where it belongs, wash your laundry and make your bed. Now the room looks cleaner than before until again you start bringing more books and things, and again the system disintegrates and becomes disorganized. To keep things in order requires constant energy input.

So entropy is the degree of disorder or randomness in any system. The second law of thermodynamics says that entropy increases with time. It reflects the instability of a system over a period of time if there is nothing to stabilise it.

In human relationships, we have interactions day after day and these relationships also become higgledy - piggledy. We let things build up in our inner chambers. These inner chambers become more and more disorganized as we store more and more, just like the books and clothes in our room. We keep harbouring things, and one day what we harbour explodes, unless we do something about it. We need input to stabilise any relationship to iron out the wrinkles or differences, so that we don't harbour and store things forever.

But do we have to do this every time we make a mistake? Do we have to offer another person ice cream or candy to always pacify them ? This would mean a constant investment to maintain a relationship.

When constant input is required every time there is a fight or an argument with a friend or family member, you will require greater input each time. You may even have to buy them a Mercedes one day, if you can afford it at the same time. It is our business to love each other, whatever the cost. You will get hurt in the process, no doubt, and there will be a lot of energy consumption from your side, but if you are prepared for it the relationship will improve.

In a family, if you have to tolerate each other, then constant input is required. In situations where you have to give constant emotional input it is a broken family, even though you may be together.

In contrast, when there is love amongst all and when acceptance is there, then you do not have to go on offering ice cream or going to some paradise vacation spot to patch things up. It is taken for granted that you accept each other with love. The conclusion is that it is the love that you have in your heart that is the input that stablilized relationships. Things are okay. There is a greater level of acceptance.

I am not talking about tolerance. Tolerance may be a great virtue, but when you feel, "I can' t tolerate this person's mistakes", love will iron out everything, so that it is okay. From where does this love come from a pure heart; from a truthful, genuine heart.

Distrust kills a relationship, but in families where we are taught to love, to sacrifice. To accept and to remain pure, we are able to let go of everything. We can remove the incompatibility, by understanding this principle of entropy.

When the constant state of my being is love, then the need for constant input disappears and the constant input is zero. When zero input is needed, it

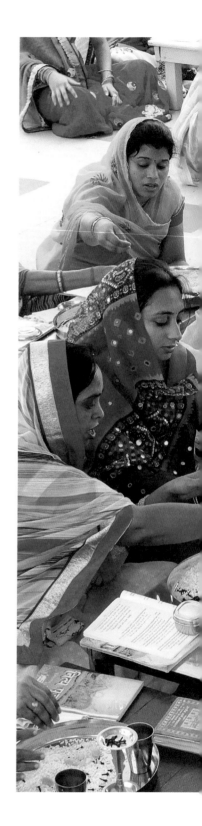

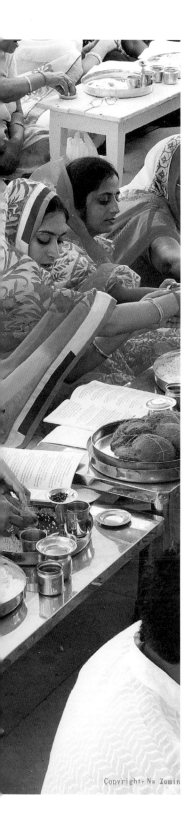

Copyright: Na Zomin

means that it is the most stable relationship, the most stable family, where I don't have to explain myself. There is no need for, "I did this because…" "I didn't want to do this because…" Where there is love, there is no need for explanations.

Marriage

Why do most love marriages fail? I think it is about time that I talked to you on this issue. Nobody guided us in those days, it was all an accident. If you ask anyone why love marriages fail, they find it very difficult to explain. They may give any number of reasons.

In the case of true love, what really happens is this: love begins and both persons' hearts expand. They accommodate anything and everything about one another. Even their mistakes become so adorable, even if she spits on you, it is so good. You will just clean your shirt or say, "Okay, let's buy a new shirt." You will not fight.

Then the next stage comes when you really start loving you start losing yourself. You start self-annihilating. You want to do everything to make the other person happy, at any cost.

But what happens when the reciprocation is not so much? The degree now starts varying and then you start judging, "Oh, I shouldn't have done this." You start retracting because you don't want to lose yourself completely. You are afraid. The fear starts out of ego. You have now started remembering yourself and the relationship now goes haywire.

You become aware of your own needs, whereas earlier you were not aware of them. You wanted to do anything and everything for the other person. Now you start realising, "Oh, I am now losing my identity. I was so-and-so, I was a musician, I was a painter,

I was a doctor but now I have to sacrifice so much."
And that is why relationships fail. The moment the
idea comes that I have sacrificed, it is the end of the
love story.

Q: Is there a solution to this? What is the most
important factor in selecting a life partner?

A: This is a very difficult question. Rather, the
answer is very difficult and what we have to implement
later is even more difficult. You have to use your heart.
From whatever I have seen so far, the little life I have
gone through, my answer is don't expect too much.
I really mean it. Sahaj Marg is all about acceptance.
And when we learn this art of accepting whatever
comes in life, whether it is a situation, circumstance,
job, business, employment or a spouse, it is the
acceptance that makes it successful. Even bacteria
can mutate to survive in a hostile atmosphere. Why
can't we? We have to constantly adapt to situations
without being disturbed. There is no perfect human
being, and if that person were perfect where would
be the need for them to be here? We are colliding
against each other with our imperfections. If we are
seeking perfection, we have to question ourselves
first: are we perfect?

Social Change

Q: As spiritual aspirants, do we also contribute to
nation building and social upliftment or do we focus
only on self - development?

A: Suppose you think of changing the entire
population of Delhi (supposing you have that ability)
but you don't change how good is it? " Let me
look after somebody else' s wife", but your wife is
struggling at home. So generosity must begin at
home, you see, with yourself first you must equip
yourself before you can help others. You have got

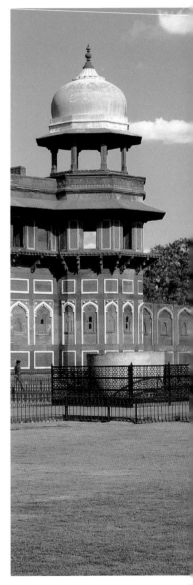

to have a million dollars before you can give somebody else a hundred thousand. If you don't have anything but you are still hoping to give somebody a million dollars, it is a pompous act. You will have to rob someone to give to someone else. When you don't have peace of mind, how can you reflect that condition to others?

There are people who create a disturbance the moment they enter the classroom. There are professors like that also you wish that this person would never come back again because of the atmosphere they carry. That is what they are. There are certain teachers you look forward to being with. There are certain friends whose association you like because of what they are.

We are moving towards perfection. Perfection in what? Not in the outer look or fancies or other things. It is the perfection in our inner balance, our inner flawless character and our manners.

I must first become perfect. I must be a balanced person inside. If, at every corner in life, at every moment, I am going to expect more and more and get dissatisfied, then I am thinking myself to be more than I am. Most dissatisfaction comes because we try to be exclusive. Exclusivity creates a lot of problems: "I want to exclusively serve the nation." Who appointed you first become perfect and then we shall see.

I would recommend that all of you read a letter that an Indian sage wrote about how to bring about world peace. In 1957, he addressed this letter to the United Nations, highlighting the method for bringing about not just the upliftment of the country but of the entire world, even the universe. Our state of balance, our condition inside, goes beyond these four walls as we progress. Its impact is galactic in scale.

Most of you will understand that what I am going to say next has nothing to do with our question, but is something by the way. What Is the formula for the velocity of light? If the distance is travelled in zero time what do you call that velocity? It is infinite velocity. Now, if Einstein's formula defines energy as being equal to mass times the speed of light squared, what happens to that energy if you insert infinity into the equation? We have all experienced it— the moment you think of transmission it is there. The energy that comes is infinite, so the source of this energy has to be infinite. Think very seriously about this. We can also prove the efficacy of the natural path scientifically.

We should not contribute anything worse to the world, at least. We try to clear the atmosphere. When we do cleaning, we are not only cleaning for our own sake, but we are contributing to the harmony in the house.

Source: From the Internet

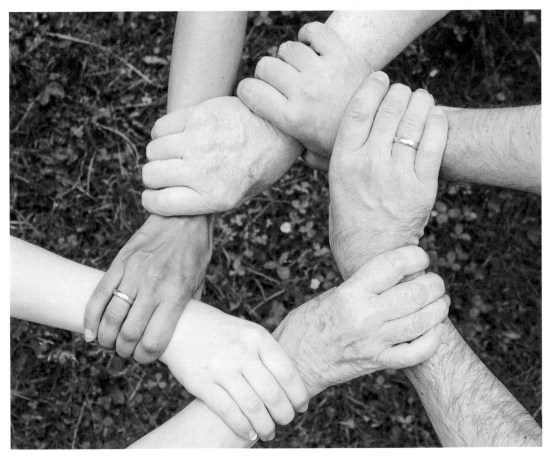

交流的艺术
The Art of Communication

交流是一个很宽泛的主题。交谈、互动、倾听、书写、肢体语言以及情感表达都是交流的一部分。

来自生活的一个场景:"亲爱的安迪,你过得怎样? 我和你妈妈很好,也很想你。请退出电脑,下楼来吃点东西吧,爱你的老爸。"

学习使用当代的交流工具与新生代交流是非常重要的。如今很多家长都无法在交流中承担自己的角色或者由于与孩子缺乏亲密感就开始一段交流,甚至开始藐视现代交流工具。这将是一个没有成功机会的想法。

交流是一件动态的事情。由于我们的时代在改变、思维在变化以及对于词汇及其含义的敏感性也在改变,所以我们必须不断地去学习如何有效、准确地沟通。保持意识、时刻学习并坚持实践,能让我们更好地掌握交流的艺术。

交流可以被大体分为言语交流与非言语交流。

言语交流实际上是一个把思想转变为语言的过程,从这个角度说,我们在有些方面可以提升得更好。

其一,掌握一门语言。掌握好一门语言,需要学习更多的词汇(正如有人所说的,一个能掌握好词汇的人是能够有效交流的),需要对该语言本土化的表达有充分的理解,还需要理解与其对应的肢体语言。

其二，避免使用与人断开连接的语言。

以下是我们常常可能说的断开连接的语言：

给他人下一些道德评判——好、坏、对、错；

给他人贴标签；

言语中暗示他人的错误以示责怪；

把自己的判断强加给他人，在谈话中用到"应该要"等词汇；

言谈中不给对方选择，会用一些"不能""必须""不得不"等词语；

表达出一些公开或隐藏的威胁。

其三，提升口语能力。很多人会问，如何提升口语能力？实际上与学习其他没有差别，就是学习、练习并增加自信，这里没

照片：王锐光摄

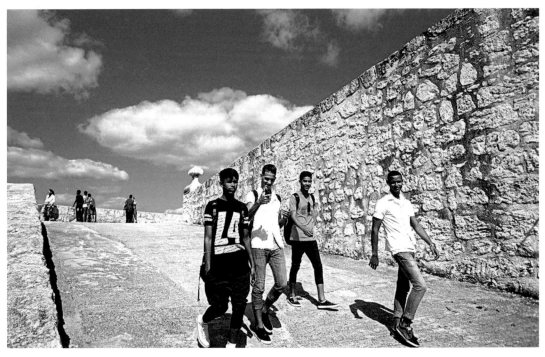

有魔法可言。比如我们可以通过阅读报纸、看该语言的电影、每次记录下一些新的单词并学习它们的用法，或者是平时多留意句子的结构等等方式来学习。

而非言语交流则从另外一个方面，在沟通中传达信息。比如，当我们与他人会面时，能穿着整洁、保持身上无异味，守时并表示出对他人的关心，那么这些已经为这次交谈奠定了很好的基础。此外，如果是一次发言，那么提前为你的听众做好准备并充分了解即将要讨论的主题，可以让你的发言更加有针对性和到位。

案例一，黑暗的阴影：我的母亲，一个无微不至的家庭主妇，经常就我父亲把外面的脏东西带回家进行教育。有一天，当我父亲到家时，发现母亲正疯狂地擦拭地板上的一个污点，并且开始对此进行"教育"："我不知道你都带进了些什么，但是我无法擦掉它们。"他花了一会工夫研究了下当时的状况，没说一句话，直接把窗台边遮挡住阳光的一个雕像移走了。就这样那个斑点瞬间消失了。

请花一点时间感受一下这个案例带给你的启发，再继续阅读后面的文字。

——有时不急于反应，而是观察、倾听，解决的办法会变得更加简单。

案例二，农场与家庭：某天下午，一名男子和他的妻子开车穿过一个郊区，他们之前刚刚大吵了一架，互相不说话。终于丈夫准备打破沉默并对他的妻子说一些讽刺的话："看农场上里的那些牛和猪，它们没有使你想起你的那些亲人吗？"妻子回答说："是的，确实是，他们让我想起了我法律上的亲属。"

请花一点时间感受一下这个案例带给你的启发，再继续阅读后面的文字。

——交谈中互相给予尊重，因为你传递出去的一定也会再回到你身上。

如果想要提升你的交流能力，那么以下有6个简单的方法可以尝试去练习：

第一，言语保持积极且表达精确。

请尝试从积极的方面与他人交谈，例如，可以告诉人们你希望做什么而不是不希望做什么，告诉别人你喜欢什么而不是不喜欢什么。

为了吸引人注意力，你的言辞必须简洁、精确且必要时需再重复一次。

确认自己的言语是否单调、独白式的以及过度传播。请避免这些事情，因为他们可能干扰听着的注意力。

第二，学会观察。

请一位朋友记录下你与别人的谈话，回放它们并尝试改善。

观察你对父母、子女、兄弟姐妹及配偶的反应，看看它们是否正是你的亲人们所做的，而你又不喜爱的行为。

第三，自我学习。

聆听一些伟大的演讲，学习如何进行演说以及如何吸引听众的注意，例如可以找一些像TED一般的简短演说，或者是总统演说以及一些纪念性演说。

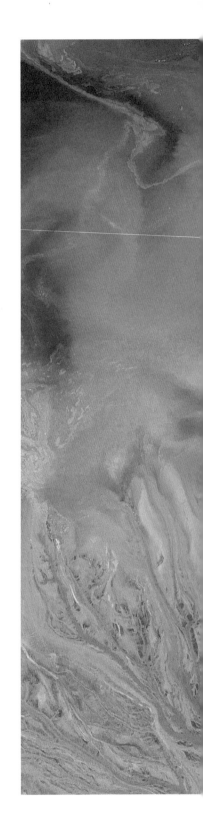

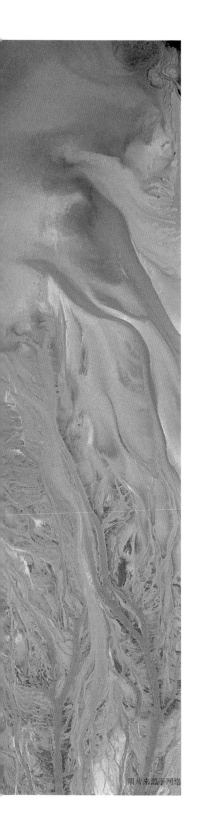

照片来源于网络

加入一些国际组织，例如头马国际演讲俱乐部（Toast Master）。

第四，更好地倾听。

仅仅成为一名好的倾听者就已经是一名好的交流者。语调、停顿和认可都是倾听的一部分。

给自己创造机会参与一些开放性的话题。

避免在谈话中与他人产生对抗与争论。

第五，随时做好准备。

在一些演讲中，我们可以通过提前做好一些准备让这次演讲更加得体。比如：

注意我们的肢体语言（保持微笑以及与他人的眼神交流）。

提交组织好交谈的内容，适当的时候讲一些故事和笑话

用一些图片、图表以及引用。

精确把控时间和信息。

第六，用心交流。

用心交流并不意味着情绪化，只是打开心扉保持真诚与谦虚的态度与他人进行交流。

在交谈的过程保持爱心并显示出对他人的关心。

这些用心的细节能够给对方留下一个好的感觉。

（根据满心资料整理）

The art of communication is a vast subject. Speaking, interacting, listening, writing, body language, emotional expressions are all part of communication.

Let's start with a daily scenario.

"Dear Andy: How have you been? Your mother and I are fine. We miss you. Please sign off your computer and come downstairs for something to eat. Love, Dad."

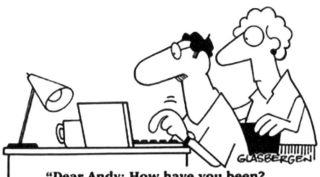

**"Dear Andy: How have you been?
Your mother and I are fine. We miss you.
Please sign off your computer and come
downstairs for something to eat. Love, Dad."**

Learning modern day tools to communicate with the new generation is very important. Many parents are unable to be present in a conversation or begin a conversation due to lack of familiarity and even developing contempt for modern tools. That would be a non-starter.

Communication is a dynamic thing. Because of the changing times, changing mindset, and changing sensitivity to words and its meaning, one has to constantly learn how to communicate effectively, precisely. So be aware of continuous evolution of consciousness. We have to learn constantly and practice too, so that we will grasp the art of communication.

Communication can be divided into verbal and non-verbal communication.

Communication requires conversion of thoughts

to a language. Form this aspect we can improve our communication.

Firstly, we need to master the language and enrich our vocabulary. It is said that the one who has a command over vocabulary would be able to communicate effectively. There is a need for a full understanding of the local expression and body language.

Secondly, we must avoid disconnecting language. Avoid these:

MORALISTIC JUDGMENT- good, bad, right, wrong

LABELS

BLAME - implying fault

NO CHOICE -"can't" "must" "have to"

DEMAND - open or hidden threat

IMPOSING MY JUDGMENT - "should" "ought"

Thirdly, we need to improve our spoken language. Many people ask how to improve our spoken language. In fact, it has no difference. One has to learn, practice and gain confidence. It is no magic. For example, we can read newspapers, watch movies, write down new words and understand its usage. Paying attention to sentence construction, learning 5 new words and its usage a day will drastically improve one's language.

Non-verbal communication is another way to convey messages. When we meet someone, we dress neatly, smell right and are punctual, which is a good foundation of our communication. When we give a speech, to prepare for the audience and have a good knowledge of the subject will make a big difference.

Case 1: Dark shadow

My mother, a meticulous housekeeper, often lectured my father about tracking dirt into the house. One day he came in to find her furiously scrubbing away at a spot on the floor and launching into a lecture. "I don't know what you've brought in," she said, "but I can't seem to get this out. "

He studied the situation for a moment and, without a word, moved a figurine on the window-sill where the sun was streaming in. The spot immediately disappeared.

Please take some time to read the case and think about it, then read the following text.

So don't react. Observe. Listen. Solutions are simpler if we observe the problems.

Case 2: Farm and family

A man and his wife were taking an afternoon drive through the countryside. They had just had a big argument and were not talking to one another. Finally the husband decided to break the silence and say something sarcastic to his wife: "Look at all the cows and pigs in the pasture. Don't they remind you of your relatives?" The wife replied, "Yes, they do. They remind me of my in-laws."

Please take some time to read the case and think about it, then read the following text.

Give respect. What goes around comes around.

If you want to improve your communication skills, you must learn 6 simple lessons.

Lesson 1 - Be Positive & Precise

Tell people what you want done and NOT what you don't want done, what you like NOT what you don't like.

To draw attention, you must be brief, precise and may confirm once.

Identify monotony, monologue and over communication.

Avoid them as it will lead to blunting the listener's attention.

Lesson 2 – Observe

Ask a friend to record your conversation with people and listen to its playback and improve.

Observe your reaction to your parents, children, siblings and spouses and see if you behave the exactly same manner as your dislike of those dear ones.

Lesson 3 – Teach yourself

Listen to great speeches and learn what and how the speaker speaks and holds the attention of the audience.

You will normally find them in short speeches like Ted, Presidential speeches and commemoration addresses.

Join Toast Masters International.

Lesson 4 – Listen Well

Intonation, pauses, acknowledgements are all part of listening.

A great listener alone can be a great communicator.

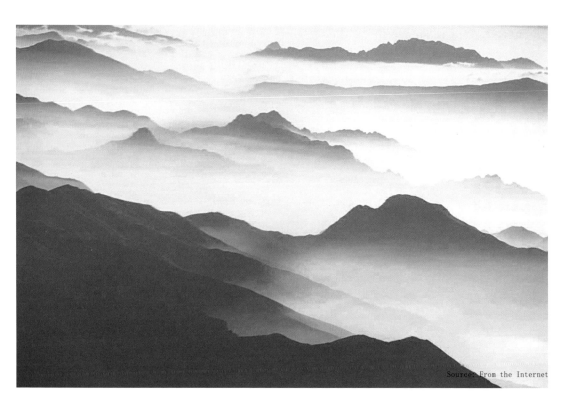

Source: From the Internet

Create opportunity to interact with open ended questions.

Avoid antagonism & argumentation.

Lesson 5 – Prepare

We can prepare in advance to make the speech more appropriate. For example:

Mind body language (Smile, Eye contact).

Be organized! Tell jokes and stories.

Have pictures, quotes and charts.

Be Precise with time and the message.

Lesson 6 – Finally Use your heart

Use the heart does not mean emotional. Just open your heart to start the communication with sincere and humbleness.

Be Caring and Concerned.

These details will leave the audience with a nice feeling.

(From Heartfulness)

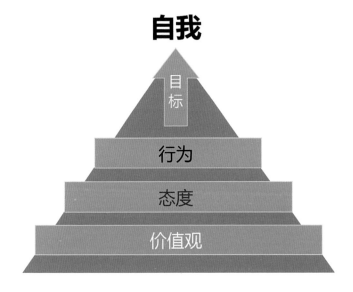

自我发展——价值观与目标
Self-development — Values and Goals

　　自我发展与成长的核心就是塑造一个良好的价值体系并将其付诸实践，这可以帮助我们平衡精神与物质生活，从而过上符合伦理的物质生活。爱因斯坦就曾说过："不要尝试成为一个成功的人，而要尝试成为一个有价值的人。"由此可见价值对于成长与生活的重要性。

　　关于自我成长有一个等式：自我成长=价值观+目标。

　　我们都有一个更高的自我，一个理想的典范以及目标，它们对我们的存在至关重要。基于真实自我的本质而产生的目标和价值观，会帮助我们形成一个良性循环，实现自我成长，并最终达到自我实现。这个良性循环就起步于一个与真实自我相协调的目标，从而产生精化的价值观、信仰和态度，它们可以帮助我们调整行为以获取来自实践的经验和知识，并最终通过练习达到完美。

　　持续地调整其中每一环的内容，可以使我们的价值观、态度以及行为保持一致，这一过程帮助我们达到自我实现这一目标。所以建立起与真实自我相协调的价值观对于个人成长和社会和谐是非常重要的。拥有正确的价值观，采取相应的行动，平凡人也可以完成非凡的事情。

　　我们将分别介绍有关价值观与设立目标这两方面的内容：

一、价值观

继续阅读前,请花一点时间思考以下问题:

(1)价值是什么?生活中是什么人或者什么因素帮助我们塑造了个人价值观以及信仰?

(2)价值观是可以被教授和习得的吗?

(3)我们天生就有价值观吗?

(4)关于价值观的学习有年龄限制吗?

你的价值观是决定你如何思考、做决定、感知以及最终行动的方向标。改变行为必须开始于检查你内在的核心价值观。自我及人本身比任务与事情更重要,而这些又比所谓的系统与概念更重要。但如果你认为事情、威望和想法比人及自我更有价值,那么你的选择和行为将会让人大跌眼镜,并且会带来悲伤、失望和失败,同样还可能伤害到你周围的人。

以下有一系列可参考的个人价值观、态度以及行为:

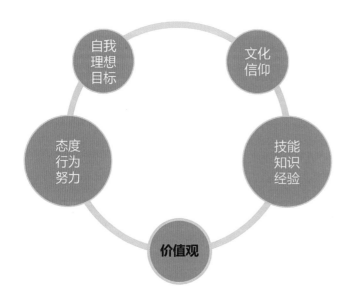

反省、道歉，即使没有错误。

目标导向。

以下有一系列可参考的有关心灵成长的价值观、态度以及行为：

诚实，把苦难当作上天的礼物。

简单、朴素。

把所有人当作上天的孩子。

对于错误的行为不要存在报复的心理。

带着感恩的念想进食。

塑造自己的生活来唤醒他人心中的爱。

睡前，为自己的错误行为沉思。

练习一——我的三个核心价值观是什么？

让我们先对比一下"对自己与他人负责"以及"以自我为中心"这两者的区别，请尝试回答以下几个问题：当我们被欺骗时有何感受？当我们欺骗他人时又有何感受？当别人的行为显得非常得体时，我们会怎么想？当我们的行为非常的得体时，他人又会如何想我们？

现在，你可以轻轻地闭上双眼，保持静默3分钟，在心中温柔地问自己："我的三个核心价值观是什么？"然后把浮现的答案在纸上记录下来。

如何建立并实践价值观？

实际上，价值观就是我们生存的原则，我们每天都基于自己的价值观做各种决定。问题是当我们建立目标和价值观时，又应该是什么原则指导我们？答案依赖于我们认为什么是重要的——野心还是抱负。

以下有一些帮助我们确立价值观的原则：

(1)决定是基于什么是好的还是什么是令人愉悦的？（什么是好的是价值观问题，而什么是令人愉悦的则出于娱乐的态度）

——锻炼还是沉溺。

——保持耐心还是保持懒惰。

(2)帮助内心成长的是价值观。

——真诚，谦逊还是不计一切代价获取胜利；自以为是以及傲慢。

——阅读、沉思、内省，冥想，帮助他人还是寻求自身的重要性，展示出来并获取关注。

(3)基于你的心灵、头脑和身体的需求而区分优先次序

——沉思、阅读和冥想还是烧饭、锻炼和看电视。

那么如何在生活中实践它们，活出这些价值观呢？

练习二——学会保持宽容、耐心和帮助

以下是一些可以帮助你做到宽容与耐心的步骤：

(1) 放弃偏见。

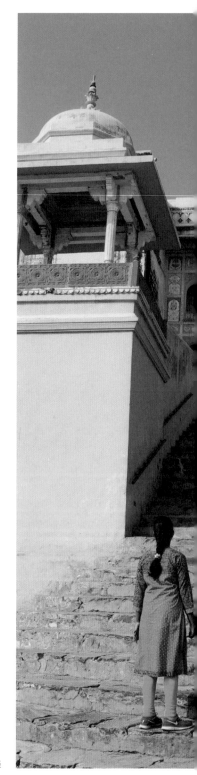

照片：那泽民摄

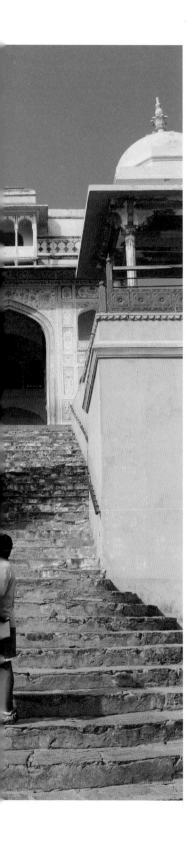

（2）学习倾听他人：耐心地倾听和了解总是比说更重要，倾听会让你知道并理解对方的感受以及他的理由。

（3）变得耐心：有些冲突并非是隔夜就能化解，无论你有多努力。事实上，有些时候越想努力去解决问题，反而会使问题更遭。其原因在于你给了它太多的注意力。要允许事情自然地恢复，之后再在正确的时候行动，而对方也需要准备好，然后顺其自然。

（4）发展和谐：在你的心中，真诚呼唤和谐，将"和谐"放在"正确"的前面。

（5）不需要去改变他人：尝试去理解他人的立场和观点，永远将别人视为比自己更伟大，这样你才会愿意去理解他们的观点，才能明白"感同身受"的含义。

（6）让自己的生气离开：有意识地让自己的生气离开，将这种境况当作成为更好的人的机会。

（7）放松并放下。

（8）不去评判。

（9）接纳并开阔自己的视野。

（10）对待别人像希望别人对待自己一样：将他人当作你的兄弟姐妹。所有的兄弟姐妹经常打架，仅仅几分钟之后，他们又会抱在一起，玩在一起。这里没有爱的遗失，你们也能这样吗？

（11）超越妒忌。

(12) 接受别人的不容忍。

(13) 柔然、关切、平衡地说话：当你说话的时候，你会发现当你的声音流平稳，没有刺耳的声音和尖锐的起伏，这会反映出你内在状态的平衡。

当生活中发生冲突、矛盾和不和谐的时候，尝试用以上的一些步骤去调整自己的内在状态与外在行为，看看是否会有什么不同。

二、目标

个人发展的良性循环就起步于一个与真实自我相协调的目标，所以目标的重要性可想而知。与此同时，当目标被设定以后，我们就有了一个清晰的方向，这会让我们充满活力与动力地行动起来，甚至有时给我们提供了一个挑战以致我们有机会跳出固有的思考模式。

问：你的目标是什么？

答：做更少的事，但是有更多的时间和金钱去做事。

大部分人都会认为目标只是一厢情愿的想法而已。然而实际上它们并不是。它们可以实现并且可以通过行动被实现得很好。问题的关键在于如何设定清晰而恰当的目标。建议以"SMARTER"为原则设定你的目标：

(1) S (Specific) ——把大而具体的目标分解成每一小步。

(2) M (Motivational) ——对于这个目标你是否有足够的激情？

(3) A (Accountable) ——可计量的，过程中你是否能衡量进步？

照片：王锐光摄

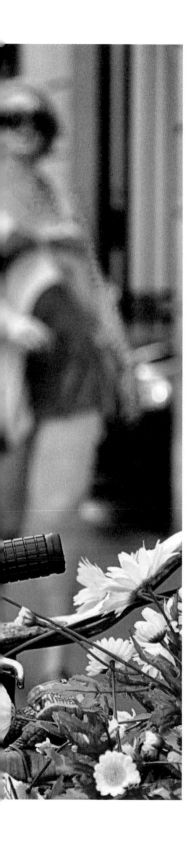

(4) R (Reachable) ——可实现性。天上不会掉馅饼, 目标的设立不是天马行空的, 必须是可实现的, 而同时也需要我们脚踏实地推进。

(5) T (Time bound) ——一个目标的设立需要有时间限制。

(6) E (Extendable) ——可扩展性。实现目标后还可延伸。

(7) R (Responsible) ——有责任心。设定目标时还需要考虑你的目标是否会影响他人。

例如, 如果一个人想要在10年内成为百万富翁, 那么他需要把这一总目标化解为具体的行动, 如何能做到, 以及考虑清楚在前进的过程中有哪些标志可以表明他在朝目标靠近。所以一个目标必须是有时间限制的, 如果没有, 那么这就不叫目标。

我们的目标也可以分为很多种, 个人的、家庭的、专业上的, 或者是心灵成长上的, 等等。

——个人目标

一些个人目标包括健康、智力、专业水平以及心灵健康, 例如:"我将在3个月内减10磅体重""我希望每周能散5次步""我希望每个月能读一本书""我希望获得硕士学位或者获取一个专业证书""我希望每周能练习一次内省 (记录下每次引起自己次优反应的事件, 并反思如何改善) "。

——专业性目标

我们拥有各自的事业，所以需要生涯目标和职业目标，这其中还包括预算，时间，收入和盈利目标。

——家庭目标

家庭是把人类聚集在一起的机构，所以家庭目标是重要的。我们可以通过与朋友和家人谈论自己的需求和目标，使他们参与其中。记录并接纳他们看法，共同使目标变得清晰可见。

——心灵目标

心灵目标的本质是抽象的，但是人都是由身、心、灵三个部分组成，所以心灵目标是必要的。有时候，灵性目标也可能需要家人的合作和参与，才能和谐地推进。

照片：那泽民摄

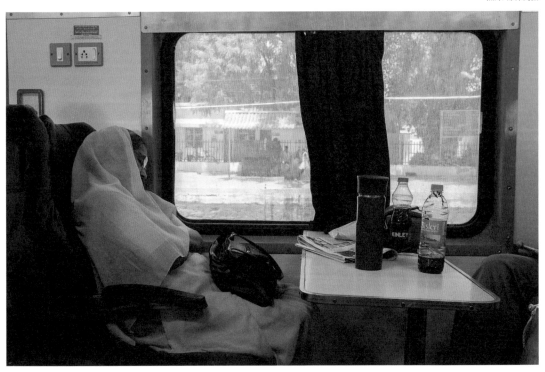

如此多类型的目标同时出现在我们的生活中,如何平衡各个目标,对于我们创造平衡、和谐的生活也是非常重要的一门艺术。为更好地保持平衡,仍然有些事情是我们可以尽力而为的:

(1) 写下并重温你的目标。创建你自己的目标列表;

(2) 确保目标之间是一致且相互支持的;

(3) 平衡好投入到各个目标之间的时间和精力;

(4) 保持耐心;

(5) 如果需要请不要害怕调整这些目标直至你依据SMARTER的原则定好目标。

有些时候,我们也会在设定目标时犯一些错误,比如,目标太大、太多且不具体,或者没有明确记录下来。请避免这些情况的出现。

千里之行始于足下,任何一棵大树都是从一颗种子的生命开始酝酿。所以请从第一小步开始,不要害怕犯错,缓慢、勇敢而坚定地去实现你的目标。但请谨记,在实现目标的过程中你仍然需要照顾好生活的各个方面。

在一个大家都奔跑而从来不走路的世界,在这个地方,我们知道所有东西的价格却忘了生活的价值,我们可以决定放慢脚步来庆祝并且提醒自己我们是什么构成的:爱、和平、真实、无暴力和正确的行为。

让我们调频我们的价值观,设定合理的目标并调整我们的行为,把焦虑转变为平和,恐惧转变成爱,战争转变成非暴力,分裂转变成正确的行为。让我们手牵手前进,这样这个世界会成为我们的家园。

练习三——行动起来

这个练习需要持续数月的时间才会看到实际的效果，你可以选择以下一个练习进行或者几个练习同时展开：

（1）基于一个价值观养成一个新的习惯（比如，学会尊重遇到的每一个人；无论遇到何种情况毅然保持微笑的面容和乐观的内心；坚持每天观察自己的内在状态和外在行为，并用记日记的方式记录下来等）。

（2）发现并改变一个习惯（比如，避免懒惰；避免逃避困难；坚持早睡早起等）。

（3）每天坚持静心冥想2次，每次10分钟（如果可以尽量在固定的时间和地点进行，那将对你帮助很大）。

（根据满心资料整理）

The core of self-development and growth is to build an aspirational set of values to live by. It will help us achieve a balanced life focused on a spiritual goal and an ethical material life. Albert Einstein once said: "Try not to become a man of success, but rather try to become a man of value." We can see the importance of values on our growth and life.

There's an equation about self-development: Self = Value + Goal.

We have the higher Self, Ideal and Goals which are central to our existence. Having a Goal that is consistent with the real Self will be a virtuous cycle. Its starts with defining a goal which is consistent with our SELF, refining your values, altering behaviors, gaining knowledge based on experience and practicing to get perfect.

Constant adjustment to align our values, attitudes, behaviors, cultural beliefs is essential to reach that pre-defined goal which we set for ourselves. The adjustment reinforces the process of reaching the Goal which ultimately reaches to self realization. Ordinary people can do extraordinary things.

We will introduce 2 parts: Values and Goal-setting.

1. Values

Please take some time to think over the following questions:

(1) What are values? What people and factors in our lives will help to shape our individual values and beliefs?

(2) Can values be taught and learnt?

(3) Are we born with them?

(4) Is there an age limit to such learning?

Your values are the anchor that determines how you think, make decisions, feel and ultimately behave. Changing behaviors must begin with examining your internal core values. If you value things, prestige or ideas more than people and self, your choices and behavior will be poor and bring sorrow, loss and failure to your life as well as hurt those around you.

A Sample Set of Personal Values, Attitudes, Behaviors:

Discipline, Prioritize, work hard

Humility, Fairness, Empathy

Kind, Generous, Giving

Honest, Truthful

Simple living

Respect, Politeness, Not hurting others

Treat others equally, avoid jealousy

Forgive and forget

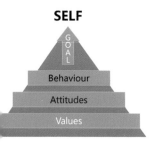

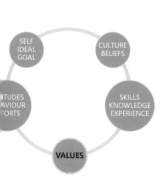

Introspect and apologize even if not wrong

Goal Oriented

A Sample Set of Spiritual Values, Attitudes, Behaviors:

Be truthful. Accept miseries as Gifts from God

Be plain and simple

Know all as children of God

Be not revengeful for wrongs done

Eat in divine thought

Mould life to rouse feeling of love in others

Bed time, repent for wrongs committed

Exercise 1: What are my three core values?

Let's compare responsibility to the self and others and self-centered. Try to answer the questions.

How do we feel when we are cheated?

How do we feel when we cheat someone else?

What do we think of others when they behave in a noble way?

What would others think of us when we behave in a noble way?

Now you can gently close your eyes and keep silent for 3 minutes. Ask yourself "What are my top three core values" and then write them down.

How to set and practice our goals?

What are the principles that should guide us when we create our Goals and Values? The answer lies in the understanding of what is important – Ambition or Aspiration.

Some principles to help us with goals and values:

(1) Decide based on what is good vs. what is pleasant? (What is good is a value and what is pleasant is entetain-ment)

——Exercising vs indulging

——Being Patient vs being lazy

(2) What helps inner growth is of value

——Sincerity, Humility vs Winning at any cost and being self righteous and arrogant

——Reading, Contemplation, Introspection, Meditation, Helping vs Seeking importance, showing off and looking for attention

(3) Prioritize based on the needs of your Soul, Mind and Body—— Thinking, Reading, Meditating vs Cooking, Exercising, Watching TV.

Exercise 2: Learn to be tolerant, patient and helpful

These are ways to help you:

(1) Give up prejudice

(2) Learn to listen to others: Listening is always more important than speaking. Listening enables you to learn and understand what another person is feeling and why.

Source: From the Internet

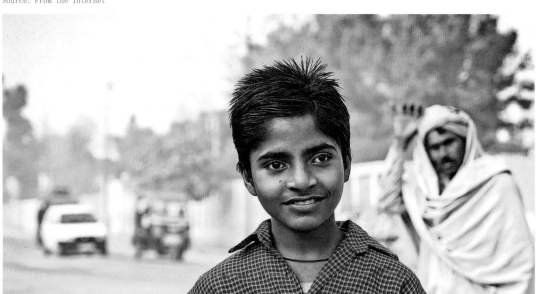

(3) Be patient: Some conflicts will not resolve overnight, no matter how much you try. In fact, sometimes trying to fix it only makes it worse because you give it too much attention. Allow things to heal naturally and then act at the appropriate time. The other person also has to be ready to let go.

(4) Develop humility: In your heart, sincerely wish for harmony. Put harmony before being right.

(5) Don't need to change others: Always see the other person as greater than yourself. Then you will try to understand their point of view; to understand means to "stand under".

(6) Let my anger pass: Consciously let go of resentment. See the situation as an opportunity to become a better person.

(7) Relax and let go

(8) Don't have to justify

(9) Accept to broaden my vision

(10) Treat others as I want them to treat me: Treat others as your brothers and sisters. Small siblings often fight, but ten minutes later they are hugging and playing, and no love is lost. Can you be like that?

(11)Transcend jealousy

(12)Accept another's intolerance

(13)Speak with softness, care and balance: When you do speak, see if your voice can flow evenly, reflecting a balanced inner state, without harshness or sharp rise and fall.

When any tension, conflicts or disharmony happen, please try to follow the above steps to adjust your inner state and external behavior, and to see if there's any difference.

Source: From the Internet

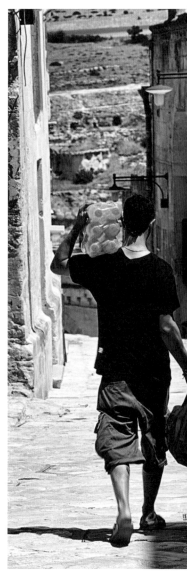

2. Goals

The virtuous cycle of self-development starts with a goal that is consistent with the real Self. At the same time, setting goals will give you direction, energize you, provide a challenge, and make you think outside the box.

Q: What are your ambitions?

A: Having less to do. And more time and money to do it.

Many think goals are about wishful thinking. But actually they are not. The goals must be realistic and well thought. The key is how to set clear and right goals. We suggest you can follow the SMATER principles.

Setting SMARTER Goals:

(1) S(Specific)——Specific and Bigger goals broken down into small steps

(2) M(Motivational)——Do you have sufficient passion

(3) A(Accountable)——Can you measure progress?

(4) R(Reachable)——Not pie in the sky

(5) T(Time bound)——Time bound

(6) E(Extendable)——Having reached the goal, extend.

(7) R(Responsible)——Does your goal affect others?

For example, if one wants to be a millionaire in 10 years, he needs to break it down as to how to get there and what the signs of getting there are. Goals must be time bound if not they are not goals.

Our goals can be divided into personal goals, professional goals, family goals and spiritual goals.

Personal Goals:

It includes making personal goals of health, mind, profession and spiritual well being. Examples: "I would like to lose 10 pounds in 3 months", "I would like to read one book a month", "I would like to go for a walk 5 times a week", "I would like to get a Master's degree or Professional certification", "I would like to practice introspection once a week (Write down incidents which resulted in sub optimal response from yourself or Introspect on how you could have improved)".

Professional Goals:

We have careers and businesses. So we need for career goals and professional goals, including Budget, time, revenue and profit goals.

Family Goals:

Family is the institution that holds the humanity together so Family goals are important. We can talk with friends and parents about the need and setting up of goals so that we can get them involved, write down and agree on them, then make the goals visible.

Spiritual Goals:

The essence of spiritual goals is abstract. All the people are physical, mental and spiritual. Spiritual goals are necessary. Spiritual goals may also involve the cooperation of one's family.

We have so many different goals in our life. How to balance all the goals is an important art of living a balanced and harmonious life. There is still something that we can do:

(1) Write and review the goals. Create your own goals worksheet

(2) Make sure the goals are consistent and mutually supportive

(3) Balance time and energy devoted to all the goals

(4) Be Patient

(5) Don't be afraid to calibrate the goals as needed till you settle down with SMARTER goals

Sometimes we will make mistakes in setting goals, such as too big, too many, or too specific goals. Please avoid these.

A thousand journey is started by taking the first step. Any big tree starts from the life of a seed.

So start slowly. Don't be afraid of mistakes. Remember to take care of all aspects of life.

In a world where everybody is running and never walking, where we know the price of everything but have forgotten the value of life, we have decided to walk in order to celebrate and remind ourselves what we are made of: Love, Peace, Truth, Non-Violence, Right-Conduct.

Let's adjust our values, goal setting and our behavior. Let's turn anxiety into peace, fear into love, war into non-violence, exclusion into right-conduct. Let's walk hand in hand so that this world turns into our home.

Exercise 3: Action now!

It will take a few months to see the effect of the practice. You can choose one or a few the following exercises to start.

(1) Create a new habit based on one Value (Ex., expecting everyone, always keep smile and be optimistic, observe your inner state and write diary).

(2) Recognize and change a habit (Ex., Avoiding laziness, avoid escaping from difficulties, Go to bed early and get up early).

(3) Meditate twice a day for 10 minutes (If you can fix your time and place, it will be more helpful).

(From Heartfulness)

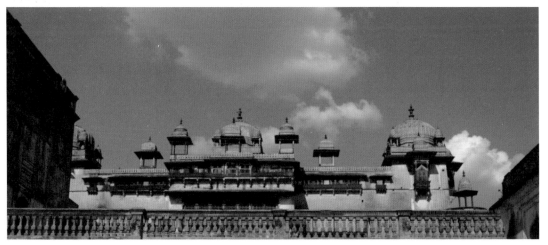

为每个人创造精神健康
Creating Mental Well-being for One and All

亲爱的朋友们：

　　我们人类的身体在观察和照料我们的健康时有一个非常奇妙的特点——当一切正常的时候，由于我们的心没有给出任何信号，我们会处于一种无忧无虑而且忽略身体健康的状态。可是当有什么不对劲的时候，心就一定会让我们知道——只要我们去聆听。

　　例如，如果我们的呼吸是健康和正常的，我们甚至都不会注意到呼吸的存在，但是假如患了感冒或哮喘，我们就一定会注意到自己的呼吸。精神健康也是如此，当一切都处于健康状态，我们甚至对自己的精神状态毫无察觉，会在内心深处感到平衡与满足。可是一旦这种平衡被打破，我们的心就会向我们发出清晰的报警信号，告诉我们有什么东西出问题了。我们

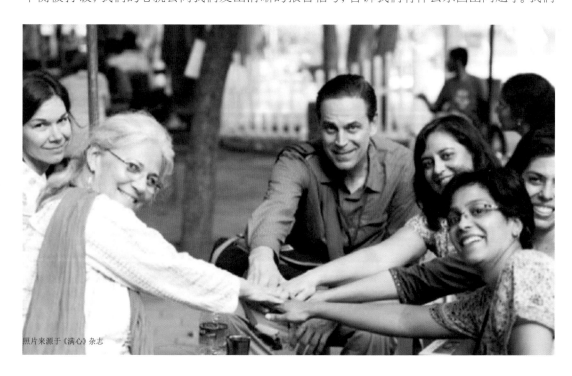

照片来源于《满心》杂志

会感到焦虑、抑郁、恐惧和愤怒，假如处理不当，这些情绪会恶化为精神疾病。

今年世界健康日的主题是抑郁，如果我们研究统计资料，其原因显而易见。根据WHO (世界卫生组织) 的资料表明，全世界超过3亿人生活在抑郁之中，而这也是在全球造成疾病与障碍的主要原因。还有，与抑郁相关的自杀是目前造成15～29岁年轻人死亡的第二位主要原因。这些统计数据让人震惊，我们正面临着全球范围的心理失衡流行病。

这有很多原因和缘由，并不是所有都能解决，但很清楚的一点是，在当今时代我们需要一些能够更好管理精神健康的基本方法。

长期以来精神疾病总是笼罩着一种耻辱，这里有一个原因。我们这个种类的名字，智人，意思是"有智慧的人"。甚至"人" (man) 这个词也来自梵文 "manas"，意思是头脑。作为一个种类，我们认同我们的头脑远远超过自己的身体。

你可以在我们日常生活的反应中看到这一点。如果有人对你说"怎么了，你的脸色看起来不太好！"那么你可能会觉得被冒犯；但如果有人说："你的脑子进水了！""你简直蠢透了。"对精神健康的一点刺激就会让我们的自尊更加受到伤害，无论针对的是我们的智商、思考能力，或者是我们的情感成熟程度。这就是为何精神疾病会比身体疾病更让人蒙羞。糖尿病比精神分裂症更让人容易接受，尽管两者都是严重的健康问题。

精神健康是一个敏感的话题！而这是可以理解的，因为事实上，自我本身就是我们精神机体之一。这些精神机体——数千年来在瑜伽中被认知为"细体"——作为人类的定义。我们的自我赋予了身份的认同感。

假如我们要去解决这个问题会怎么样？我们是否能找到一个简单的方法去照顾我们的细体，让其恢复活力、焕发精神和重新振作呢？在今天如此快节奏和高压力的世界中，有什么简单的方法能让我们重新获得精神平衡，从而让我们尽可能地感觉良好以及应付自如？我们也许无法解决所有导致精神失衡的问题，但我们至少可以尽最大的努力来照顾好自己。

四个简单的练习

以下是四个非常简单的练习，假如每天带着兴趣和热情去进行，将会对你的身心平衡有所支持和帮助。你可以在以下网址找到这些满心练习的一套三节高级研习班课程：

http://heartfulness.org/masterclass

1. 放松

学习一种简单的放松方法，能够随时随地进行。满心放松只需要几分钟，尤其有助于睡眠以及处理恐慌、压力或恐惧的时刻，或者帮助你在平时感到更知足。

无论何时当感到有恐慌或压力，你还可以使用楠迪呼吸法让自己冷静下来。用拇指按住右边鼻孔，然后用左边鼻孔进行10次深呼吸：激活副交感神经系统，让你冷静下来。

2. 冥想

冥想陶冶头脑。头脑学会柔和自然地专注于一个事物，在以心为对象的冥想中我们更加深入内心——在那

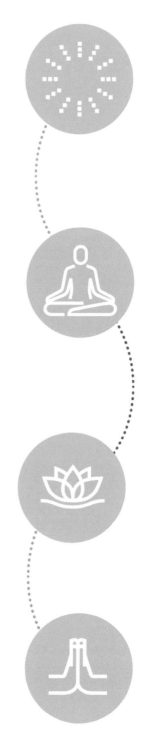

照片来源于《满心》杂志

里我们找到自己感觉、启悟、创意和爱的世界——出来时焕然一新，并带着深深的幸福感。

3．清理内心和头脑

和身体一样，你的头脑和内心也需要清理。通过保持内心和头脑的清洁，你会找到内在的宁静、轻盈、明晰和冷静。你的头脑将恢复其自然的灵活性并放下沉重的负担。

4．与更高自我的连接

要感觉到整体和连接，我们需要滋养三种机体——身体、头脑及心灵。我们可以通过与内在更高本我的连接，从而滋养我们的头脑和心灵。这种连接通过古老的祈祷练习而建立。祈祷在心中制造出能够感受到爱的内在状态。祈祷带我们进入内心的无限世界，那里充满如此多的喜悦和美好。

遵循自然的周期

除了进行以上的练习，精神健康还有赖于尽可能自然的生活方式。人类是自然的一部分，因此每天、每周、每月以及更长的周期会连接到我们的生理机能。例如，我们每天有活动、休息和睡眠的周期，假如我们与这些周期相反，这就像逆流而上——我们的健康会受损，尤其随着我们的年龄增长。与月亮周期一致，我们还有每月的周期。同样，假如我们与这些不协调，我们将会逆流而上。

这里有四个帖士帮助我们与自然协调一致，并能更好地照顾自己。

1．夜晚安眠

尽量在晚上10点前睡觉，这样你能获得睡眠时间的最大收益。在睡觉前，花些时间放缓节奏并放松，或者享受陪伴家人和朋友，而不是看电视或玩电子游戏，这些活动会刺激大脑并导致睡眠不安。

2. 做早起的鸟儿

早起冥想，让你带着内在连接、平衡的感觉在一天中有个美好的开始。假如你能带着这种内在状态进入一天的活动，你就能处理面前的任何事情，无论有多大的挑战。

3. 以爱说话

当我们醒着的时候，大部分时间都用于与其他人沟通。那么话语尽量友善、温和以及适度，这会改变你的生命。要学习更多如何做到的内容，请浏览以下网址：

http://www.heartfulnessmagazine.com/speak-with-love/.

4. 以爱进食

当我们清醒的时候，花很多时间去做的另一样事情是进食。进食和消化食物带来能量。为了身体和精神的健康，我们需要花些时间进食，以便我们的能量储备可以专注于消化。我们在进食的时候一边走路、驾车、看电视或者坐在电脑前，这样可能吗？不行！身体正在转移能量去进行其他任务，因此我们的消化系统会加重负担。我们很多人已经失去了进食的艺术。

那么，这就有如何进食的问题。我们对所吃的食物心怀感恩吗？如今科学研究表明感恩在任何行动中的益处，而怀着感激、爱以及悲悯的态度进食，比起贪婪或者缺乏意识地进食，对我们的身体会有十分不同的效果。为什么不用这个方式去关爱我们的身体呢？长远来看，这会产生巨大的收益，并且有很多研究都将抑郁和肠道健康联系在一起。

所以，亲爱的朋友们，我们的精神健康值得去滋养。我很乐意回答任何关于这个重要的健康领域的问题，并希望你能尝试为这个目的而设计的满心练习。通过这些练习，我们学习聆听自己的心，并照顾自己以及他人。

满心能够把我们带到最开始的基础——精神平衡和平静的状态。从那里开始，我们可以扩展更多、更多，为了体验内在喜悦和启悟的状态，这是我们人类与生俱来的权利。请加入我们吧。

你可以发送电子邮件给我：daaji@heartfulness.org，访问我们的网页：www.heartfulness.org以及daaji.org，并在我们的满心点或者通过智能手机的冥想吧（Let's Meditate）应用程式自行体验满心练习。

祝一切顺利！

达济

照片来源于《满心》杂志

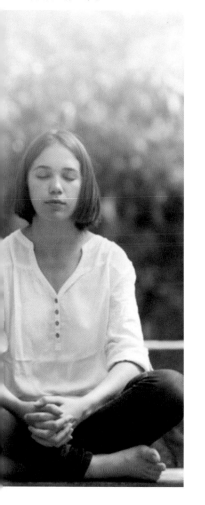

Dear friends,

Our human system has a very wonderful characteristic when it comes to observing and looking after our health – when nothing is wrong, we remain carefree and oblivious to our health, as our heart does not give us any signals. But when something is wrong it definitely lets us know – as long as we listen to it!

For example, if our breathing is healthy and normal, we are not even aware that we are breathing, but if we have a cold or asthma, we will surely be aware of our breathing. The same is true with our mental well-being: when everything is healthy, we are not even aware of our mental processes, and we feel balanced and contented within ourselves. But when things are out of balance, our heart gives us clear warning signals that something is wrong. We feel anxious, depressed, fearful or angry, and these emotions can escalate into mental illness if not managed properly.

The theme for World Health Day this year is depression, and the reason is clear if we examine the statistics. According to the WHO, more than 300 million people are now living with depression, and it is the leading cause of ill health and disability worldwide. Also, depression-related suicide is now the second leading cause of deaths for 15 to 29 year-olds. These statistics are chilling. We are facing an epidemic of mental imbalance around the world.

There are many reasons and causes, and not all of these can be solved, but one thing is clear: we need some basic tools to better manage our mental well-being in this day and age.

There has long been a stigma around mental illness, and there is a reason for that. Our species name, Homo sapiens, means "wise man". Even the word "man" comes from the Sanskrit word "manas"

Source: From the Internet

meaning mind. As a species, we identify with our mind much more than with our physical body.

This you can see in our everyday reactions. If someone tells you, "What is wrong, your face looks terrible?" you may be offended, but you will be more offended if they say, "You have lost your mind," or "You are so dumb!" Our ego is hurt more by a slight to our mental well-being, whether it be to our intelligence, our thinking capacity or our emotional maturity. That is also why mental illness is much more of a stigma than physical illness. Diabetes is more acceptable than schizophrenia, even though both are serious health problems.

Mental health is a sensitive subject! And, it is very understandable, actually, as the ego is itself one of our mental bodies. These "mental bodies" — known for thousands of years as the "subtle bodies" in Yoga — define us as human beings. Our ego gives us our sense of identity.

So what if we focus on trying to solve the problem? What if we can find simple ways and methods to look after our mental bodies so that they are refreshed, rejuvenated and revitalized? What simple tools can help us regain mental balance, so that we can feel as good as possible and function well in today's world of high stress and fast pace? We may not be able to solve all the issues that lead to mental imbalance, but we can at least do the best we can to look after ourselves.

FOUR SIMPLE PRACTICES:

Here are four very simple practices that, if done daily with interest and enthusiasm, will support and help to balance your mental well-being. You will find a set of three masterclasses on these Heartfulness practices at http://heartfulness.org/masterclass.

1. RELAX

Learn a simple relaxation technique that you can do anywhere, anytime. The Heartfulness Relaxation takes just a few minutes and is especially helpful when you need to sleep, deal with moments of panic, stress or fear, or to generally help you to feel more contented.

You can also use nadi breathing to calm yourself down, whenever you feel panicked or stressed. Hold your right nostril with your thumb and take 10 deep breaths in and out through your left nostril: it actives the parasympathetic nervous system, which calms you down.

2. MEDITATE

Meditation regulates the mind. The mind learns to gently and naturally focus on one thing, and in heart-based meditation we go deeper into the heart – where we discover our world of feelings, inspiration, creativity and love – and come out refreshed, with a deep sense of well-being.

3. CLEAN YOUR HEART AND MIND

Your mind and heart need to be cleaned just like your body. By keeping them clean, you will find inner stillness, lightness, clarity and calm. Your mind will regain its natural flexibility and let go of its heavy burden.

4. CONNECT WITH YOUR HIGHER SELF

To feel whole and contented, we need to nurture all our three bodies – the physical, mental and spiritual. We can nurture the mental and spiritual bodies by connecting with our higher Self within the heart. This connection is done through the time-honored practice of prayer. Prayer creates that inner condition in the heart that can be filled with love. Prayer takes us into the infinite world of the heart, which is filled with so much joy and beauty.

BE IN TUNE WITH NATURAL CYCLES:

As well as doing the above practices, mental well-being depends on living as natural a lifestyle as possible. Human beings are part of Nature, and

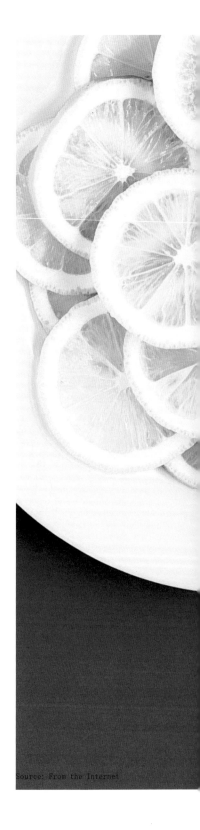

Source: From the Internet

244

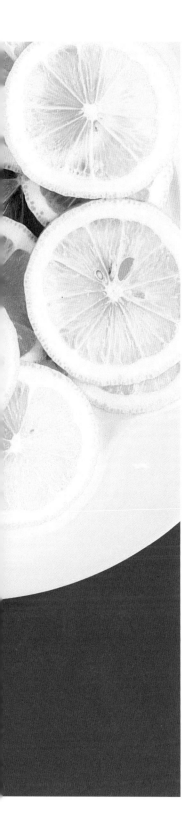

as such have daily, weekly, monthly and longer-term cycles that are wired into our physiology. For example, we have daily cycles of activity, rest and sleep, and if we go against these it is like swimming upstream – our health is badly affected, especially as we age. We also have monthly cycles that are in tune with the lunar cycles. Again, if we are not in tune with these, we will be swimming upstream.

Here are four tips that help us fine-tune with Nature and look after ourselves better:

1. GET A GOOD NIGHT'S SLEEP

Try to sleep by 10 p.m. so that you are maximizing the benefits of your sleeping hours. Before sleeping, spend some time winding down and relaxing, or enjoying the company of family and friends, rather than watching TV or playing video games, which over-stimulate the brain and lead to restless sleep.

2. BE AN EARLY BIRD

Wake early and meditate. This gives you a great start to the day with a contented, balanced feeling inside. And if you can carry that inner state with you out into your day, you will be able to handle anything that is thrown at you, no matter how challenging.

3. SPEAK WITH LOVE

When we are awake, much of our time is spent in communicating with others. So make an effort to speak gently, tenderly and moderately; it will change your life. To learn more about how to do this, visit:

http://www.heartfulnessmagazine.com/speak-with-love/.

4. EAT WITH LOVE

The other thing we spend a lot of time doing while we are awake is eating. Eating and digesting food takes energy. To be healthy, both physically and mentally, we need to take time to eat, so that our energy reserves can focus on digesting. Is that possible when we are eating on the go, driving, watching TV, or sitting at a computer screen working? No! The body is diverting energy to the other tasks being performed, so our digestion suffers. Many of us have lost the art of eating.

Then, there is the matter of how we eat. Are we grateful for what we are eating? Scientific studies are now showing the benefits of gratitude in any activity, and eating with an attitude of gratitude, love and compassion has a very different effect on our bodies than eating with greed, or a lack of awareness. Why not take care of our bodies in this way? It will pay great dividends in the long run, and there are many studies now linking depression with gut health.

So dear friends, our mental well-being is worth nurturing. I would be happy to answer any questions you have about this vital area of health, and hope you will try the Heartfulness practices that have been designed for this very purpose. Through them, we learn to listen to our heart and care for ourselves and for others as well.

Heartfulness can bring us to first base – to a state of mental balance and peace. From there we can take it much, much further, in order to experience the inner states of joy and inspiration that are our human birthright. Please join us.

You can write to me at daaji@heartfulness.org, visit our websites at www.heartfulness.org and daaji.org, and try Heartfulness practices for yourself at one of our HeartSpots or via our LetsMeditate App for smartphones.

All the best,

Daaji

在任何体系中获得成功的秘密
The Secret of Success of any System

我在实验与错误中花费了50年，才意识到我的妈妈，尽管连最基本的教育都没有接触过，却是绝对正确的。这在后面会详细提到，其开始是一个问题。

在任何体系中获得成功的秘密是什么?

这有一个公式:

$$成功 = f\left(\frac{外部的整合}{内部的解体}\right)$$

外部的整合: 一个将组织、任何系统与其环境进行整合的一个方法。没有任何系统、个人、家庭、生意或国家存在于真空之中。

我们的市场占有率、利润幅度、重复销售、EVA、ROI、每股营利等指标用作衡量外部整合。当我们指向个人，我们通过地位、收入、进入管理层的速度等作为其职业成功的反映，来计算他们的外部整合。对于一个国家来说，决定性的因素在于支付平衡，每位公民的平均收入、贸易状况和经济增长。相同的概念，不同的衡量形式。

内部的解体是指在组织内部引起的所有争斗: 流言、误解，在背后捅刀子以及对工作的失望和离职等，还有内部解体的其他表现形式。在我们的个人生活中，内部的分裂是我们头脑中产生所有困惑的一种功能。自我疑惑，自我贬低和不信任，以及我们其他一些最具破坏性的行为。在一个国家中分裂的标志是社会中经常引起的歧视，常态化的冲突，不论是性别、信仰、宗教、民族或肤色等方面。

问题是，为何这个公式可以预言成功？从物理学中我们获悉能量是固定的。我们发现在每一个系统中固定的能量都在以一种可预见的方式进行分配。它首先要处理内部的不融合，剩余的部分才会来到外部的整合。举例来说，如果你正在生病，处在四分五裂的状态，那么你用于讨论和如何把控变化的市场的力量就会很弱。

在一家公司中充斥着内部的不融合，大多数的能量流向了对个人背后的保护，保护一个人在政治上或管理上的权力，伴随着在系统中的一席之地。例如一位经理去参加他本来不想参加的委员会议，目的是在于保护自己的利益。

所以，需要的是进行较少的内部整合，当这个目标达到，

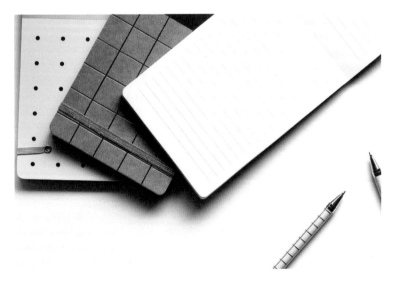

Source: From the Internet

就会有更多的能量进入到外部的整合中去,从而就会有大得多的机会在一个体系中获得成功。但是,内部的解体意味着什么?让我们从它的反面来理解。如何将内部的解体最小化?通过整合。

什么是整合?什么是整合化的组织?一个健康的系统。整合是健康的同义词,是疾病的反义词。我们如何去形容一个心智健康的人?他是一个完整的人。我们如何去形容一个身体上甚至在精神上都有病的人,他或她是破碎的。对生病的家庭和生病的社会来说也是一样,破碎,解体。

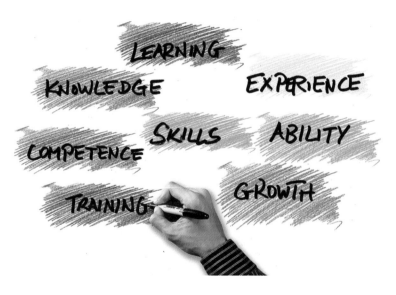

所以,现在成功的秘密是什么?并非外部的整合,那是获得成功的结果,那是产出。我们需要明白是什么造就了成功,那就是要认出投入的价值。

成功是内部的整合,也就是说,健康。当我们与同伴道别的时候,我们不都是对那个人心存某种希望吗?在全世界所有的语言中不是都说,祝愿健康吗?当我们拿起酒杯,不都是在相互祝愿"祝你快乐""祝你健康""为了你的健康干杯"吗? 不同的语言都是表达出同样的意思。

拥有很多财产, 其价值何在? 或者说, 如果我们生病了, 还有哪种成功能够用来衡量我们? 那个时候你最想做的可能是交出自己所有的财产, 来换取再次的健康。真正成功的秘密在于你到底有多健康, 你的个人; 你的家庭; 你的生意; 你的国家。

聚焦于你的组织的健康以及如何整合, 你的子系统有多么平衡。利润就是一个指标, 衡量你在平衡投入的方面有多完美。它就是网球比赛上的记分牌, 它告诉你玩得有多好。但一直注视记分牌而忽视球, 并不能帮助你赢得比赛。重点是在于关注比赛, 而结果会积极地写在记分牌上。

所以管理的作用是什么? 对于首领、家长或是国家领导人来说? 就是让他们在管理、领导或是照顾的系统去争取成为并且保持健康。

我的妈妈, 无论何时我告诉她, 我在我的客户, 或在我的著作上取得了某些难以置信的成功时, 她总会叹口气说, "最重要的是你的健康。"这就好像是在说, 你告诉我你的成功这很好, 可是儿子, 最重要的是你的健康。

谢谢妈妈。想你!

真诚地!

伊贾格·爱迪斯 博士
行政总裁/主席 爱迪斯学院
www.ichakadizes.com
www.adizes.com

It took me fifty years of trial and error to realise that my mother, who did not have even an elementary education, was absolutely right. More about that later. But it starts with a question. What is the secret of success of any system? There is a formula:

$$\text{success} = f\left(\frac{\text{External Integration}}{\text{Internal Disntegration}}\right)$$

External integration is the way in which the organisation, any system, is integrated with its environment. No system, person, family, business or country exists in a vacuum.

We measure external integration in business by market share, profit margins, repeat sales, EVA, ROI, earnings per share, etc. When we refer to individuals, we calculate external integration by their career success as reflected in status, earnings, or rate of ascending in the hierarchy of the organisation. For a nation the determining factors are balance of payments, average income per citizen, trade conditions and economic growth. Same concept, different forms of measurement.

Internal disintegration is all the internal fighting that occurs in organisations: the rumours, misunderstandings, back stabbings, frustrations with the job and turnover of people, among other manifestations of disintegration. In our personal life, internal disintegration is a function of all the confusion in our head: the self-doubt, self-disrespect and mistrust coupled with some of our most destructive behaviour. In a nation the disintegration is marked by a society where discrimination frequently occurs and where confrontations are the norm, whether in terms of gender, creed, religion, nationality or colour.

The question is: why does this formula predict success? We know from physics that energy is fixed. I discovered that the fixed energy is allocated in a predictable way in every system. It moves first to deal with internal disintegration and only then does the surplus overflow to external integration. For example, if you are ill and falling apart you will have little energy available to discuss, plan or organise how to handle the changing market.

In a company riddled with internal disintegration, most of the energy is dedicated towards protecting one's back, preserving one's political and managerial power, along with a place in the system. For instance, a manager decides to sit in committee meetings he does not want to attend in order to protect his interests.

So what is wanted is less internal disintegration. When that occurs there is more energy available for external integration and much greater opportunity for success of the system. But what does internal disintegration mean? Let us understand it through its opposite. How do you minimise internal disintegration? By integration.

Integration is synonymous with health and disintegration with sickness. What do we say about a mentally healthy individual? He is all together. What do we say about a physically or even mentally sick person? He or she is falling apart. Same for a sick family or a sick country. Falling apart. Disintegrating.

So, now, what is the secret of success? Not external integration. That is the result of having success. That is the

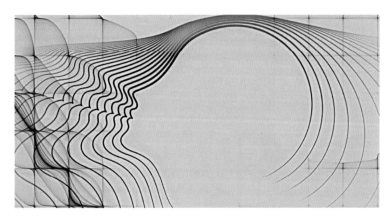

照片来源于《满心》杂志

output. We need to understand what makes success? Which is to recognise the value of the input.

Success is internal integration i.e. being healthy. Don't we say in all languages, "Be well", when we wish something for the other person as we part company? Don't we raise a glass and wish each other "*Na zdravlje*", "*Salud*", "To your health": the same expression in different languages.

What is the value of having a lot of possessions, or whatever success we might measure ourselves by, if we are sick? Have you ever been very sick? You were probably most willing to surrender all your possessions just to become healthy again. The real secret of success resides in how healthy you are. You personally, your family, your business, your country.

Focus on the health of your organisation and how integrated it is, how aligned the subsystems are. Profits are a measurement of how well you have perfected aligning the inputs. It is the scoring board of the tennis match. It tells you how well you played. Focusing on the scoring board and ignoring the balls will not help you win the game. The point rather is to focus on the game, which in turn reflects positively on the scoring board.

So, what is the role of management? Of leadership? Of a parent? Of a national leader? To make and keep the system they are managing, or leading, or parenting, healthy.

My mother, whenever I would tell her about some incredible success I had with a client or with my book, would sigh and say, "*Ha ikar ha bruit* (What is most important is your health)," as if to say, it is nice all you are telling me about your success, but watch it son. What is really most important is your health.

Thank you mom. Just thinking.

Sincerely,

Dr. Ichak Kalderon Adizes

CEO/President,

Adizes Institute

www.ichakadizes.com

www.adizes.com

满心练习
Heartfulness Practices

满心放松

找一个舒适的坐姿坐下，轻轻地闭上双眼。

挪动一下脚趾。

感觉来自地球母亲的能量流入自己的脚趾。去观察它放松的效果。

让这个能量上升，流向自己的双脚和脚踝，感觉它如何让身体的这个部位放松、恢复。

让这个能量向上来到小腿，感觉它带来的放松效果，小腿肌肉放松，膝盖，大腿，触及椅子的整个部位，包括背部，感觉这个能量在放松整个背部。

让这个能量向前移动，放松腹部的肌肉，胸腔，肩膀。尤其在这里感觉融化的作用、放松的作用，在自己的肩膀上，感觉都在融化。

让这个能量流向胳膊，感觉手臂肌肉的放松，手肘、手腕、手掌、手指以及指尖。让这个能量流入并放松整个手臂。让这个能量通过指尖慢慢流出。

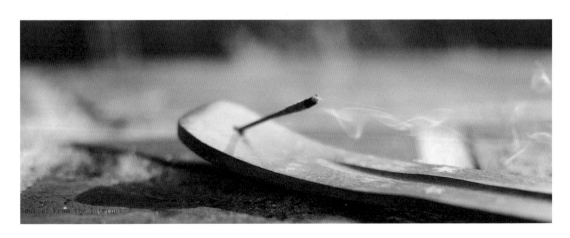

把注意力转向颈部的肌肉，去感觉这个能量在使颈部所有的肌肉放松。让这个能量向上，放松所有的脸部肌肉，额头，眼睛，嘴唇，耳垂，头顶。感觉这个能量以非常柔和的方式从脚部逐渐向上升，经过刚才的步骤一直到头顶。如果想回到身体依然绷紧的某个部位，现在可以去特别留意，直到那个部位全然放松。

扫描一下整个身体，从脚趾到头顶。

将注意力转向心，在那里停留一阵，感觉沉浸在内心的爱和光之中。

保持静止和平静，慢慢沉浸于自己的内在。

只要愿意，尽可能久地停留其中，直到自己愿意从这个状态中出来。

满心冥想

轻轻地闭上双眼并放松。

将注意力转向内在，并在此瞬间观察自己。然后，轻轻地假设光之源已经存在心中，从内照亮并吸引着自己。一缕神圣的光。

以轻柔及自然的方式进行，不必专注集中。假如发现自己思维分散，请轻轻地回到内心之光的意念上。

沉浸于内心的光，让自己沉浸其中。保持静止和平静，只要愿意，尽可能久地停留其中，直到自己愿意从这个状态中出来。

满心清心

轻轻地闭上双眼并放松。

现在把注意力放在背部，从头顶到尾椎。

想象日间所有的杂质和不净物都从这里离开。只是暗示一切在发生。

从哪里离开？从背部排出，想象从头顶到尾椎的整个背部。

如何离开？想象以烟雾的形式离开。

维持这个过程。

在这个状态上稳定下来后，可以加速这个过程。

进行15～20分钟。然后在清心的过程中轻轻加入下一个元素。想象有光从上面降下，由前面进入自己的身体。穿过整个身体，从背后出去并帮助移除杂质和不净物。光填补移除杂质和不净物之后所留下的真空。最后，坚定地暗示自己：所有的杂质和不净物都被移除，感觉自己非常简单和纯洁。

满心临睡冥想

轻轻地闭上双眼并放松，非常轻柔地将注意力转向心。

想象"已经存在心中的光之源将我的注意力转向内在，从内在吸引着我的注意力"。

如果有杂念升起，轻轻地提醒自己正在冥想，以光之源冥想。

把注意力停留在心中，感觉心中对合一以及自己所能达到的至高的渴望。唤醒最深处的本我进行指引，尽量深入内在。

Heartfulness Relaxation

Sit comfortably. Gently close your eyes.

Wiggle your toes.

Feel the energy entering into your toes from Mother Earth. See its relaxing effect.

Let this energy move upward to your feet and ankles. Feel how it rejuvenates and

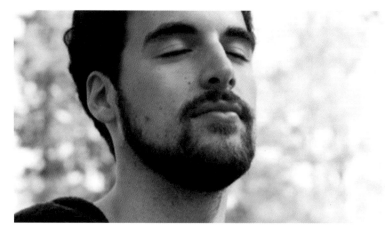
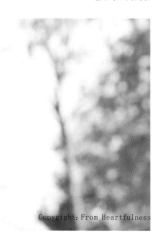

relaxes this part of the body.

Let this energy move upward to your lower legs. Feel the relaxing effect of this energy moving upward to your calf muscles ... your knees ... your upper legs ... and the entire area touching the chair, including the back. Feel this energy relaxing the entire back.

Let this energy move forward relaxing the abdominal muscles ... the chest area ... your shoulders. Here especially feel the melting effect, the de-tensioning effect, in your shoulders. Feel that they are melting away.

Let this energy move to your arms, feeling its effect though your biceps ... and elbows ... your wrist area, your palms, ngers and fingertips. Let this energy move and rejuvenate the entire length of your arms. Let this energy ooze out through your fingertips.

Pay attention to the neck muscles. Feel the energy relaxing all the neck muscles.

Let this energy move upward, relaxing all the facial muscles ... forehead ... your eyes ... lips ... earlobes ... the top of your head.

Feel this energy now flowing in a very gentle way from the feet, rising slowly upward through the steps we just followed, to the crown of your head.

If you feel like revisiting a stressed area of your body, you can pay extra attention there now until that part of the body is also fully relaxed.

Then scan the whole system now from toe to top.

Move your attention to your heart. Rest there for a little while. Feel immersed in the love and light in your heart.

Remain still and quiet, and slowly become absorbed in yourself.

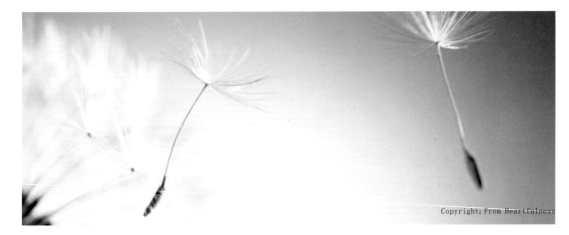

Remain absorbed for as long as you want, until you feel ready to come out.

Heartfulness meditation

Gently close your eyes and relax.

Turn your attention inwards and take a moment to observe yourself. Make a gentle suggestion that the source of light already present in your heart is illuminating it from within and drawing you in.

Do this in a gentle and natural way. There is no need to concentrate. If you find your awareness drifting to other thoughts, gently come back to the idea of the light in your heart.

Feel immersed in the light in your heart, and let yourself become absorbed.

Remaining still and quiet, rest there for as long as you want, until you feel ready to come out.

Heartfulness cleaning

Close your eyes very gently and relax.

Now focus on your back, from the top of the head to the tailbone.

Think that all the complexities and impurities from the day are going away. It is a suggestion that it is happening.

From where? Out your back, from the top of the head to the tailbone. Imagine it. How? Think that they are going in the form of smoke.

Continue with this process.

When you have settled with this, then accelerate the process.

Do this for 15 to 20 minutes.

Then gently add the next element to the cleaning process. Imagine that the light is descending from above and is entering from the front side of your system. It is passing through your entire body, going out from the back and helping you to remove those complexities and impurities.

This light is filling up the vacuum left by the removal of complexities and impurities.

At the end, make a firm suggestion: all the complexities and impurities are now removed, and I feel a lot simpler and purer.

Heartfulness bedtime meditation

Close your eyes and relax, with your attention drawn very gently towards the heart.

Think that "The source of light which is already present inside my heart is drawing my attention inward, it is pulling my attention inward."

If thoughts do arise, gently remind yourself that we are in meditation, meditating on the source of light.

Rest your attention in the heart, feel the longing that is there in the heart to be one, and the highest you can be. Call upon this deepest Self for guidance. Try to go deeper within.

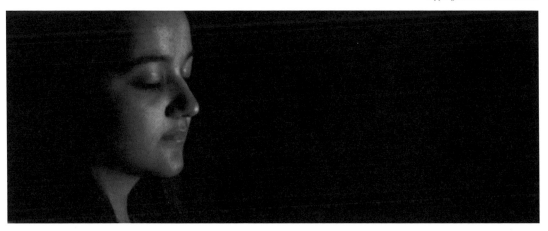

有关葛木雷什·D. 巴特尔

为人熟知爱称为达济, 葛木雷什·D. 巴特尔是满心冥想的第4任向导。他曾多次发表演说并已成为典范, 供寻求东方的心和西方的头脑完美融合的朋友效法学习。他曾周游世界, 能够畅通无阻地与来自各种背景和社会各界的人士交流互动, 他尤其关注当今的青少年。

他是一位多产的演讲者和作者, 您可以在下网站 (www.daaji.org) 阅读他最近的文章。

About Kamelesh D. Patel

Known to many as Daaji, Kamlesh D. Patel is the fourth spiritual Guide in the Heartfulness tradition of meditation. He is a role model for students of spirituality who seek that perfect blend of eastern heart and western mind. He travels extensively and is at home with people from all backgrounds and walks of life, giving special attention to the youth of today.

He is a prolific speaker and writer, and you can read his latest writings at www.daaji.org.

后 记

心，可以引领我们走过这一生。但是是如何的光明可以带我们圆满地度过此生？这是值得我们探讨的人生议题。

我们时常需要唤醒内在的精神。满心的冥想、清心以及内在沉思的方法可以帮我们调整，每个人都可以活出内在的精神健康。

"艺术与心灵成长"是一门自2012年就在同济大学开设的通识课程。在课堂上，我们可以让自己的身体完全地放松，偶尔让自己闭上双眼，忘记呼吸，深入内在，而感受到地球母亲的疗愈力量。在这门课中，我们还会用到色、声、香、味、触法，让学生可以深入内在，观察内心。意识到那些沮丧，那些焦虑，甚至低落的情绪，不是我们原本的状态。完全可以通过自己，唤醒内在的精神状态。

希望通过此书，我们慢慢会找到内在的爱，内在的智慧，内在的正能量，然后非常积极地去面对生活中的各种经历，甚至会觉得痛苦是非常美妙的礼物，只是它的包装看似有些不太好看。

此书得以出版，特别感谢葛木雷什·D.巴特尔 (Kamlesh D. Patel) 大师的智慧，他的真知灼见和充满爱的指引将带领大家编织自己的命运。同时，感谢印度Heartfulness团队和中国满心翻译团队，以中英两种文本呈献给大家。在本书的编辑过程中，感谢同济大学出版社那泽民编审一如既往的支持，感谢我的研究生沈文成的编排与设计。

最后，再次感谢所有启发我、给予我灵感的人。

俞鹰

2020年5月于同济大学

Postscript

Heart can lead us through this life. But how can light bring us through this life? This is an issue worthy of our discussion.

We need to awaken the inner spirit. Meditation, cleaning and inner prayer can help us adjust, and everyone can live a mental health life.

Art and Spiritual Growth is a general education course at Tongji University since 2012. In this class, we can relax our bodies completely, occasionally allow ourselves to close eyes, forget the breathe, go deep inside, and feel the healing power of mother earth. We will also use colors, sound, smell, taste and touch to enable students to go deep inside and observe themselves. We will realize that black mood, anxiety and even depression are not our original state of mind. We can fully awaken the inner state of mind by ourselves.

I hope through this book, readers will gradually find inner love, wisdom and positive energy. Then they can positively face all kinds of experiences in life, even recognize that pain is a wonderful gift that looks bad.

This book benefited from the wisdom of Kamlesh D. Patel. His thoughtfulness and his loving guidance can help us design our own destiny. I greatly appreciate the help of the people who have been directly involved in the editing of this book, including the Indian Heartfulness Team, the Chinese Heartfulness Translation Team, Editor NA Zemin from Tongji University Press and Art Editor - my MA student SHEN Wencheng.

Again, I would like to thank all those who inspired and enlightened me.

YU Ying
At Tongji University
May 2020

图书在版编目（CIP）数据

艺术与心灵成长：汉、英／俞鹰主编．-- 上海：
同济大学出版社，2020.11
ISBN 978-7-5608-9513-0

Ⅰ．①艺… Ⅱ．①俞… Ⅲ．①艺术—应用—精神疗法
—研究—汉、英 Ⅳ．① R749.055
中国版本图书馆 CIP 数据核字 (2020) 第 176481 号

中华文化创意丛书
艺术与心灵成长

主　　编　俞　鹰
责任编辑　那泽民
装帧设计　润泽书坊＋沈文成＋刘烨
责任校对　徐春莲
出版发行　同济大学出版社
　　　　　（地址：上海市四平路 1239 号　邮编：200092　电话：021-65985622）
网　　址　www.tongjipress.com.cn
经　　销　全国各地新华书店
印　　刷　上海丽佳制版印刷有限公司
开　　本　720mm×1000mm　1/16
印　　张　16.5
字　　数　330000
版　　次　2020 年 11 月第 1 版
印　　次　2020 年 11 月第 1 次印刷
书　　号　ISBN 978-7-5608-9513-0
定　　价　128.00 元